D0500186

# BLIND
# FAITH

# BLIND FAITH

The Unholy Alliance of
Religion and Medicine

RICHARD P. SLOAN, PH.D.

St. Martin's Press  New York

This book is dedicated to the memory of
Jean and Seymour Sloan, whose antinomic amalgam
of sweetness and acidity informs every page.

www.stmartins.com

Library of Congress Cataloging-in-Publication Data

Sloan, Richard, Ph. D.
    Blind faith : the unholy alliance of religion and medicine / Richard Sloan. — 1st ed.
        p. cm.
    Includes bibliographical references and index.
    ISBN-13: 978-0-312-34881-6
    ISBN-10: 0-312-34881-9
    1. Medicine—Religious aspects. I. Title.

BL65.M4S56 2006
201'.661—dc22

2006046218

First Edition: November 2006

10  9  8  7  6  5  4  3  2  1

# CONTENTS

# ACKNOWLEDGMENTS

As in all things great and small in my life, this book being no exception, Jessie Gruman has played a pivotal role. Hearing me grouse about the persistent and uncritical media characterizations of the beneficial effects of religious involvement despite what I perceived as the poor quality of the evidence, Jessie gently but directly encouraged me to stop complaining and do something about it. Thus began what is approaching a ten-year effort to examine the empirical, ethical, practical, and theological considerations raised by attempts to link religion and health.

Spurred by this encouragement, I asked two remarkable friends and colleagues, biostatistician Emilia Bagiella and psychiatrist and ethicist Tia Powell, to work with me to review this voluminous and extraordinarily heterogeneous literature. This two-year effort culminated in a 1999 *Lancet* publication on "Religion, Spirituality, and Medicine." *Lancet* editor Pia Pini was especially helpful working with us on this manuscript.

I remember with fondness the intellectual challenges of our next paper, "Should Physicians Prescribe Religious Activities?" Coauthors the Rev. Larry VandeCreek, Chaplain Margot Hover, and Carlo Casalone, S.J., contributed significantly not only to the paper but also to my continuing education in religious matters.

A substantial portion of *Blind Faith* was completed while I was in residence at the Bellagio Study and Conference Center of the Rockefeller Foundation, a remarkable facility providing a rich and supportive environment in a magnificent setting. While there and since, I have benefited from conversations with and the constructive criticism of fellow Bellagio scholars David Nathan, Cecilia Vicuña, Kathy Fennelly, Gabor Borit, Nick Cummings, and Alice and Warren Ilchman.

Over the years, my work in this area has been enhanced immensely by discussions with colleagues and friends Ken Gorfinkle, Don Kornfeld, the Rev. Raymond Lawrence, Peter Shapiro, Catherine Monk, Paula McKinley, Robert Pollack, John Truman, Rita Charon, Bernard Gross, Rabbi Mordechai Schnaidman, Danny Pine, and Chaplain Bonnie Olson. William Stubing of the Greenwall Foundation and Brownie Anderson of the Association of American Medical Colleges provided support to gather important information about the medical school curriculum. Journalists Jeff Sharlet, Bob Abernathy, Tom Rosenstiel, Krista Tippett, and Gary Schwitzer helped me think through the role of the media in the increased interest in religion and health.

Vartan Gregorian and Daniel Fox have given me advice and enthusiastic encouragement throughout the writing of *Blind Faith*. Henry Heffernan, S.J., helped me consider many of the theological issues that arise in this area. And I have been aided immeasurably by the opportunity to discuss these matters with my father-in-law, the Rev. Larry Gruman.

Editor Julian Zuckerbrot helped to develop the original book proposal. Mollie Glick, my agent, deserves special credit for her work in shaping the proposal that led to a contract with St. Martin's Press, and Michael Flamini, my editor at St. Martin's, took the manuscript and made it a book. I thank each of them.

# PART ONE

Religion and Health, Yesterday and Today

# 1

## INTRODUCTION

On February 22, 2004, the *CBS Sunday Morning* news program broadcast a segment about a Colorado orthopedic surgeon who prays with his patients. When does he pray with them? Not several weeks prior to surgery, for example, in an office visit when the decision to proceed with surgery is made. Not several days prior to surgery, during routine prehospitalization medical tests. Not even several hours prior to surgery. *The surgeon "asks" if it's "okay" to say a prayer when patients are gowned and on the gurney ready to go into surgery.* Put yourself in the patient's position. Would you feel free to say no to a physician dressed in surgical scrubs who is about to have your medical future in his hands, who is about to take a scalpel to your body? He could simply pray *for* his patients and do so in private. That's something that undoubtedly is quite common and laudable. But he doesn't. This surgeon prays *with* his patients.

Welcome to the brave new world of religion and health, where science, medicine, faith, and ethics exist together in a potentially explosive mixture. Although this may be a rather dramatic illustration of how religion has found its way into clinical medicine, it's extreme only by degree. In the first decade of this twenty-first century, we confront a deluge of interest in connecting religion to medicine. Dr. Dale Matthews of Georgetown University recommends that clinicians ask "What can I do to support your faith or religious commitment?" when patients respond favorably to questions about whether religion or faith is "helpful" in dealing with their illness. Dr. Matthews has also declared that the future of medicine is "prayer and Prozac." This is just the tip of an iceberg that threatens the scientific practice of medicine. Physician Walter Larimore writes that excluding God from a medical consultation is a form of malpractice. Presumably, if a doctor failed to ask questions about the presence of the Almighty in one's life, he or she could be sued. Dr. Christina Puchalski of George Washington University is one of many physicians who recommend conducting a *spiritual history* during the initial visit and then annually thereafter. In one of the most bizarrely inappropriate instances of religious influence on medical research, the U.S. National Institutes of Health is funding a research study on the impact of distant, intercessory prayer for the treatment of glioblastoma, a cancer of the brain.

The cover story of the November 10, 2003, issue of *Newsweek* magazine was entitled "God and Health." Its subtitle was "Is Religion Good Medicine? Why Science Is Starting to Believe." The subtitle is accurate. Scientists, along with the general public, are starting to believe that religion is good for your health. But the issue is not as clearcut as it might seem. The evidence about the health benefits of religious involvement is much more questionable than the popular media suggest, and there are many other problems associated with bringing religion into clinical medicine. *Blind Faith* is about the emergence of this movement and the problems—scientific, ethical, practical, and theological—that arise from attempts to link medicine with religion.

Problems notwithstanding, this belief is growing, and we can find evidence of its strength within organized medicine and among the general public. Within the medical community, considerable interest in religion exists. In December 2005, the Harvard Medical School offered a continuing medical education course called "Spirituality and Healing in Medicine." In it, the students were taught about the medical benefits of prayer and how to integrate it into medical practice. The course subtitle was "The Importance of the Integration of Mind/Body Practices and Prayer." One year earlier, the Mayo Clinic College of Medicine organized a research conference entitled "Spirituality Measured: Capturing the Elusive Effect." In November 2005, the University of North Dakota School of Medicine and Health Sciences offered a lecture entitled "Faith, Prayer and Miracles: The Role of Spirituality in the Modern Practice of Medicine." Prestigious universities have established centers devoted to exploring the relationship between religion and medicine. The George Washington University Medical School has founded the George Washington Institute on Spirituality and Health (GWISH). The Duke University Medical Center operates the Center for Spirituality, Theology and Health. The University of Minnesota has a similar organization, the Center for Spirituality & Healing. Undoubtedly, there are many more.

Within medicine, a field called *neurotheology* has arisen to study the neurobiological basis of religion and spirituality. Researchers in this field claim that by using neuroimaging techniques while someone is meditating or praying, they can take a picture of God. That is, they believe that scanning the brain during meditation or prayer yields some fundamental insights into the religious experience and, moreover, that this research bridges the gap between science and religion.

Over half of U.S. medical schools now include in their curricula courses on religion, spirituality, and health. Harvard physician Herbert Benson writes that faith in God has a health-promoting effect. Physicians David Larson and Dale Matthews argue for spiritual and religious interventions in medical practice, hope that the "wall of separation" between medicine and religion will be torn down, and, as we saw, assert that "the medicine of the future is going to be prayer and Prozac." The Christian Medical and Dental Association even trains physicians in how to evangelize in their medical practices. Doctors are encouraged to use "faith flags," rhetorical probes to determine how receptive their patients are to evangelical efforts. These are followed by telling "faith stories," narrative tales of religious or biblical principles that are relevant to the physician's life. Finally, the doctor is encouraged to evangelize overtly. The medical practice is a perfect setting to "cultivate," "sow," and then "harvest" converts.

This increased spiritual interest within the medical community has begun to produce a burgeoning scientific literature examining links between religion, spirituality, and health outcomes. Dr. Harold Koenig and colleagues report that more than 1,400 scientific papers on the topic exist. In previous papers, Koenig claimed that there were more than 850 papers on religious involvement and mental health, with more than two-thirds showing an advantage to the religiously active, and more than 350 papers on religious involvement and physical health, with more than half showing an advantage to the religious. An earlier claim asserted the existence of 325 studies in the area, of which more than 75 percent showed benefits of religious involvement.

Books on the topic appear by the dozen. Some are written by New Age gurus like Deepak Chopra and Doreen Virtue, who write about quantum healing and angel medicine. Others come from more reputable academic researchers. Koenig has been especially productive, publishing *Is Religion Good for Your Health?*, *The Healing Power of Faith*, and *The Link Between Religion and Health*. Along with Drs. Michael McCullough and David Larson, Koenig is author of the voluminous *Handbook of Religion and Health*. Other popular books in the field include *The Faith Factor* by Dale Matthews, *God, Faith, and Health* by Jeff Levin, and *Faith and Health*, a collection edited by Thomas Plante and Allen Sherman.

Given the current degree of religious involvement in the United States, the media and the general public also are intensely interested in the possible connection between religion and health. According to the Gallup Poll's Web site, American religious involvement is substantial and highly stable: 84 percent of those surveyed in 1965 believed in

God. In 1999 it was 86 percent, and in 2004 it was 81 percent. A different index of religious involvement—attendance at church or synagogue—also reveals this stability. For the period from 1992 to 2005, those who reported that they attended church or synagogue once per week was steady in the 28 to 36 percent range. For those reporting attendance almost every week, the range was 9 to 14 percent. A 1996 poll of one thousand U.S. adults found that 79 percent of the respondents believed that spiritual faith can help people recover from disease, and 63 percent believed that physicians should talk to patients about spiritual faith. Biomedical researcher David Eisenberg and colleagues noted, in a widely cited article on unconventional therapies, that 25 percent of all respondents reported using prayer as medical therapy. Some survey data suggest that patients would welcome discussions of religious matters with their physicians.

The American media also are in on the rush to find a link between religion and health. Recent articles in such American national newspapers as the *Atlanta Constitution, The Washington Post,* the *Chicago Tribune,* and *USA Today* have reported that religion can be good for your health. *Prevention* magazine has featured articles about "how religious faith can make you almost invulnerable to disease" and how "asking someone to 'say a little prayer' for you might help you heal." Other popular press articles examine the issue more generally. The cover story of the August 29–September 5, 2005, issue of *Newsweek* magazine addressed spirituality in America. The December 20, 2004, cover story of *U.S. News & World Report* was devoted to the power of prayer. A March 2003 cover story in *Parade* magazine reported on the same topic.

It is tempting to suggest that this effort to more closely link religious activities with medicine is principally the work of religious fundamentalists. Certainly, some of the proponents hold such fundamentalist beliefs. Family physician Walter Larimore, who recommends that God not be excluded from clinical medicine, is affiliated with the evangelical Christian organization Focus on the Family. Evangelical physician

Dale Matthews, another advocate of linking religion and health, also falls in this category. Their attempts to more closely connect religion and medicine very likely derive from their fundamentalist views. But to suggest that this movement is largely based on the efforts of religious fundamentalists would be incorrect. There also are a great many proponents who cannot be called fundamentalists. Physician Daniel Sulmasy is a Franciscan brother but generally takes a liberal perspective on the matter. Dr. Christina Puchalski of GWISH supports inquiries into spiritual matters by physicians because she believes the practice to be central to delivering high-quality medicine. Dr. Herbert Benson, a longtime proponent of linking religion and medicine, is generally liberal in his views about religion. In these times of increasing religious influence across all aspects of American life, interest within medicine crosses the fundamentalist/liberal dichotomy.

## VOICES OF CONCERN

Despite the remarkable and widespread popularity of the idea that religious devotion is good for your health, some voices within the scientific, medical, and religious communities have expressed caution about attempts to link religion, spirituality, and medicine in a closer bond. In recent years, several prominent scientists have written about the dangers they see in these connections. Steven Weinberg, the Nobel Prize–winning physicist at the University of Texas, and zoologist Richard Dawkins of Oxford University have produced withering critiques of religious interference with scientific inquiry. The late Stephen Jay Gould of Harvard University published a more moderate examination of the issue, essentially declaring religion and science to be two independent and nonoverlapping domains. The New York Academy of Sciences published the proceedings of a conference decrying the current flight from reason, with several contributions describing how religion contributes to this flight. Recent efforts to promote "intelligent design" as an alternative to Darwinian evolutionary theory have intensified concerns about the role of religion in science and about the low level of scientific literacy in the U.S.

Within medicine specifically, researchers and clinicians have expressed apprehension, even alarm, at this trend. I'm among those writers who have published papers that question the quality of the evidence claiming to demonstrate associations between religious involvement and beneficial health outcomes. Our papers also address the serious ethical problems that may arise if religious and medical concerns are commingled in the context of clinical medicine. University of Kentucky psychiatrist Neil Scheurich calls for a separation of "church and medicine" similar to the "separation of church and state," endorsing "a medicine that neither exalts nor demeans religious belief, but rather situates the latter among the countless values persons may hold." That is, Scheurich argues that religion is no less important, but no more important, than any other value a patient may hold. In a thoughtful critique of studies of distant, intercessory prayer that is relevant to the much larger enterprise of testing the health benefits of religious involvement, Dr. Joseph Chibnall and colleagues identify significant scientific and theological problems.

Still others have expressed alarm that scientific studies of the relationship between religion and health come perilously close to attempting to validate the tenets of religion using the tools of science. In his compelling book, *Seduced by Science,* Steven Goldberg of Georgetown University's Law Center writes about the increasing trend to subject religious doctrine and belief to scientific examination, arguing that to do so demeans religion. Indeed, nothing could be more trivializing of religion than for it to require marketing in the form of claims that it prevents disease and enhances recovery. In Goldberg's view, these efforts make religion no different from other cultural institutions of our time.

Finally, the theological community also has raised objections. The Reverend Joe Baroody has criticized how proponents of a connection between religion and medicine misuse the term *faith*, presenting it as a one-dimensional index defined by a religious activity, such as attending church. Baroody makes the especially interesting point that the thrust of the religion-medicine literature suggests that religiosity is thought to operate in the direction of improving health but that faith, in a more complex fashion, may not always work to this end. Chaplains Thomas O'Connor and Elizabeth Meakes raise questions about the qualifications of physicians to discuss religious and spiritual issues, contrasting the extremely limited exposure to these matters in medical school with the extensive training that health care chaplains receive. Writing from the perspective of social justice, Henry Heffernan, S.J., makes the important point that studies attempting to connect religious involvement with health typically fail to consider the importance of low socioeconomic status as a factor in accounting for poor health.

*Blind Faith* is a critical examination of the science, ethics, and health care policy associated with this movement. It proposes to answer three questions:

1. Do the efforts to link religion and health represent good science?
2. Do they represent good medicine?
3. Do they represent good religion?

As we will see, for most of the studies that claim to support the health benefits of religious involvement, there are serious concerns about the research methods used, raising questions about whether it is possible to draw any firm conclusions from them. The examples presented above, especially the Colorado surgeon who prays with his patients just prior to surgery, reveal that efforts to closely link religion and the practice of medicine bring with them numerous ethical considerations. Is the quality of medicine improved by these efforts? And finally, as the latter part of *Blind Faith* will make clear, there are substantial reasons to be cautious about the impact of these efforts on religion itself. What, for example, does it mean for religion to attempt to validate its tenets using the methods of science?

There may be intense current interest in the possible connection between religion and health, but this is not a new phenomenon. From the earliest societies to the present, religion and health have been intimately connected. Often they have been linked to magic, too. The Egyptians, the Greeks and the Romans, and the early Christian societies, for example, had views of medicine and health that were intimately connected to their beliefs in the supernatural. With the advent of modern science, beginning in the Enlightenment, the role that religion played in matters of medicine was diminished. But as you can tell from the polling data and the trend in our current medicine, it has not disappeared.

The most recent interest in linking religion and medicine arose in part, as Chapter 3 will show, as the culmination of a series of societal changes in the U.S. beginning with the cold war competition with the Soviet Union. Indeed, over the past fifty years, there has been a remarkable evolution of public views about science and medicine, moving from enormous levels of support to uncertainty about the scientific and medical enterprises. This change has been paralleled by a substantial reduction in skepticism and an increase in the willingness of the general public to accept statements based more on the strength of conviction than the quality of the evidence. A legacy of the New Age movement of the latter part of the twentieth century, the reverence for the subjective as a source of the truth has supplanted the reliance on objective reality, according to social critic Wendy Kaminer. Some of the support for an alliance between religion and medicine comes from this transformation.

There are other factors, too, that have set the stage for the emergence of this field. The transformation of medical practice, including an increasing reliance on high-technology medicine and changes in health care financing, has led to widespread dissatisfaction with contemporary medical care. These changes have come at the cost of human relationships in clinical care, leading to a willingness to seek other ways to provide satisfying interpersonal interactions in medicine.

Advocacy foundations have been active for many years now in promoting connections between religion and medicine. Much of the research reviewed in this book has been supported by foundations with an active interest in advancing the case that religion is good for your health. That, of course, is what remains to be determined, not what we should assume from the outset to be true.

The broadcast and print media, increasingly influenced by the profit-driven pursuit of ratings, routinely report heartrending stories about how seemingly intractable medical conditions were reversed by religious devotion, without adequately examining whether these stories are true and without presenting alternative accounts of them. Finally, interest in religion in the U.S. has gone through historical cycles, increasing and decreasing on a regular basis. Most evidence suggests that we are currently in a period of rising interest. These factors likely are the most important contributors to the current interest in religion and health. They are examined in much greater detail in Chapter 4.

Of course, one of the central considerations in this entire field is the quality of the evidence that emerges from the increasing number of research studies that have been published in the past several decades. Part 2 of *Blind Faith*, "Reading the Evidence," is composed of five chapters that examine the methods used to study connections between religion and health and the findings of these studies. It provides an overview of how science operates as well as some hints that will allow you to consider the validity of claims about the research findings that appear with increasing frequency in the media. And we'll critically examine the evidence itself. Are there really more than 1,400 scientific papers on the topic, and do the vast majority of them demonstrate a health advantage to the religiously active?

Some of this material on research methods—the essential characteristics of an experiment, how observational studies are necessary but unfortunately limited means to study many of the interesting and important research questions we have, the threats to valid scientific inferences—may already be familiar to you. If so, skip over it. But

"Reading the Evidence" also contains some very practical information on how to determine the relative merits of competing scientific claims as well as characteristics of poor-quality research studies. In a field that is characterized, unfortunately, by a great many poorly conducted studies, knowing these characteristics can help you work through the claims about the evidence.

As important as the quality of the evidence is, in some respects it is far less significant than other issues raised by efforts to link religion and medicine. Part 3 of *Blind Faith* addresses matters not related to evidence. The first of these are the ethical concerns that arise in connection with attempts to introduce religion into clinical medicine. We'll examine them in great detail later, but to anticipate, keep in mind something that we all know about dealing with doctors: that patients may be fearful and in pain and, as a result, in a subordinate and vulnerable position. Most of us have already had this experience, and it's only a matter of time for the rest of us. The resultant power that doctors have over patients increases the possibility of manipulating our religious beliefs and creating other ethical abuses.

There are purely practical problems that arise, too, when doctors bring religion into the office. These problems revolve around the increasingly limited amount of time doctors can spend with patients. These days, physicians complain loudly and often about how little time they have to spend on direct patient care. Bringing discussions of religious matters into the clinical interaction can be time consuming. Given the limited amount of time doctors can spend with patients, will they have to forgo discussion of pressing medical matters if they spend time on religious ones? Will discussions about exercise or depression be pushed aside so that inquiries about spiritual histories can be conducted? Can this problem be resolved in an acceptable manner?

And there is the matter of patient demand for bringing religion into medicine, something that the advocates believe is substantial. In this regard, as in so many others in this field, the situation is considerably more complex than it seems. In part, the complexity is due to differences in the way patient demand is measured. In part it is due to collecting data from different regions of the country and from different types of patients. Hospitalized elderly patients may have different views about discussing religion with their physicians than young patients during an office visit. Opinions may depend on whether patients are asked merely about their preferences for having discussions about religion and spirituality with their doctors in general, or asked more specifically if they want to bring religion and spirituality into clinical medicine, even if that means that they won't be able to discuss certain important medical matters.

Beyond these empirical and practical matters, there is another concern that for some may be most important of all: the impact that attempts to bring religion into the "laboratory" of the scientist will have on religion itself. Theologians have long cautioned against "putting God to the test," and we'd be hard-pressed to argue that some of the studies that appear in the literature do anything but that. Is there a danger that in doing so, that in successfully demonstrating a relationship between religious involvement and better health, the advocates will win the battle and lose the war? Will God and religion be reduced from a philosophy of how to live one's life morally and ethically, one that answers questions about the mysteries of existence, to a treatment option that appears on a health insurance plan or an over-the-counter product available in the aisles of our local pharmacy?

# 2

## RELIGION AND MEDICINE IN HISTORY

**Medicine and religion have been intimately connected** throughout history, and in most eras they have been connected to magic, too. Throughout, they all have attempted to answer the same basic questions. One of these is "What causes illness?" A related question is "Why did I get sick?" Of course, the answers to these and other questions vary from era to era, from civilization to civilization. But regardless of the answers, the questions persist, even to this very day. In this chapter, we briefly review the relationship between religion and medicine from early societies to the present. As the French like to say, the more things change, the more they remain the same. Despite substantial differences over the millennia, some common themes emerge.

Keep in mind that in a single chapter, it is impossible to do justice to the history of these relationships. Scholars spend their entire lives studying them, and the most we can hope for here is to frame the issue so that we can make sense of the current state of affairs.

In this chapter, we'll begin by considering religion and medicine, such as they were, in the earliest, preliterate societies. From there, we'll proceed to ancient Egypt and Judaism, then on to the Roman Empire, then finally to Christianity. From there, we'll consider the relationship between religion and medicine as the Renaissance and the Enlightenment progressed, culminating in the development of modern science and medicine among many other accomplishments.

## THE EARLIEST SOCIETIES

In the preliterate societies that preceded the Egyptian era, there were few distinctions between religion, medicine, and magic. Illness was generally seen as the product of demons or spiritual forces that entered the person, taking over vital functions, ultimately producing the disease's characteristic symptoms. Correspondingly, treatments were directed at these "causes," just as today's medical treatments address the bacteria or viruses we consider causes. If illness was the product of demonic forces that had possessed a person, they would have to be removed. In the medicine of preliterate societies, dances, incantations, sacrifices, and other rituals were performed, usually by shamans. Their aim was to rid the patient of these invading demons.

But even in these primitive and preliterate societies, there was some recognition that some ailments were caused by more mundane agents. Some stomach ailments, for example, were understood to be the product of eating certain foods. They were treated by family members or herbalists. Even in these cases, however, elements of magical treatment were present. These magical practices were used to make sure that the more prosaic treatments were effective.

## ANCIENT EGYPT

To understand the Egyptian view of religion and medicine, we need to appreciate two essential features of ancient Egyptian society. First, religions were *polytheistic,* i.e., there were many gods instead of a single one; and second, the idea of the "good" in society was a state of harmony with the divine.

Thus, illness created a state of *disharmony* with the gods, of which there were a great many. Intruding spirits sent by the gods but also by the dead or by one's enemies caused disease. To treat the disease, the intruding spirit must be removed. In the case of spirits from the dead or from enemies, magical rituals were the appropriate treatment. In the case of spirits from the gods, only a god could remove them.

Thus, an Egyptian suffering from an illness could seek the services of many different types of healers. Some of these healers were priests. Others used magical treatments. Some even used approaches like surgery and drugs. Despite the existence of these multiple approaches, they were not entirely distinct but overlapped to a considerable degree. In both the earliest societies and in ancient Egypt, medicine and health were linked not to a formal religion in the modern sense but rather to a system of supernatural causes. Treatments of disease varied widely, but in most cases they were directed at these gods or demons.

## ANCIENT JUDAISM

The key feature that distinguished Judaism from ancient Egypt and other Near Eastern cultures was monotheism: there was only one God. Another key distinction was the relationship between moral failure and illness. In Judaism, this was a central feature. In ancient Egypt, it was not. In the Old Testament, Adam's sin allowed evil, including illness, into a previously perfect world. Faithfulness to God was associated with health and prosperity. Lack of faith led to illness. Thus, ancient Judaism heralded a concern that still confronts us today: the moral responsibility for illness.

In Egyptian societies and in earlier ones, magic played an important role in the treatment of illness, but it was proscribed in Judaism.

Instead, prayer was the principal form of treatment. This makes sense, considering that the source of illness was thought to be a failure of faithfulness to God. It also is consistent with the fact that until exposure to the scientific medicine of Greece in the second century B.C., Judaism lacked a counterpart to the priests of ancient Egypt. Prayer by individuals does not require assistance.

## THE MEDICINE OF ANCIENT GREECE

It shouldn't be surprising that in a society as complex as that of ancient Greece, there was no single view of the relationship between religion and medicine. As in polytheistic Egypt, the many gods played a significant role in health and illness as well as in all other aspects of life. In the *Iliad,* for example, the god Apollo causes the death of Queen Niobe because of the excessive pride she displays in comparing herself to Apollo's mother, Leto. Disease was the result of divine displeasure at human conduct. Treatment required that the gods be appeased, usually by sacrifice or purification.

At about the same time, another view of disease also existed: diseases were the products of possession by a god or power rather than merely sent by a god. To treat this kind of possession, a "physician" sought to purify the patient, using, for example, herbs, exorcisms, or charms.

In about the fifth century B.C., one approach to medicine in Greece began to become more scientific in the modern sense. That is, Greek physicians attempted to explain illness in terms of natural, as opposed to divine or supernatural, causes. This is the tradition of Hippocrates: not only were diseases seen as the products of natural events, but this view was accompanied by an attempt to develop a systematic body of knowledge based on observation. Case histories were written, symptoms described, effects of treatments recorded. In this sense, Hippocrates founded what we call "clinical observation" today.

Hippocrates also developed what may have been the first widely accepted theory of disease. The four basic elements—earth, air, fire, and water—were associated with the four humors of the body: black bile, yellow bile, blood, and phlegm. Disease, in Hippocrates' view, consisted of an imbalance of these humors. By today's standards, of course, this theory is primitive, but judged by the standards of its own time, it was quite an achievement. Its accomplishment lay in the fact that it sought to account for disease as part of a comprehensive theory about relationships between elements of the human body and elements of the universe. The fact that it seems nonsensical today should not diminish our appreciation of how advanced it was in its own time.

Existing alongside this developing Greek rational medicine was the popular religious medicine, in which patients appealed for healing from the gods, not physicians. Although initially there were many gods of healing, the god Asclepius became the most prominent. Shrines to Asclepius were established throughout the Mediterranean. The tradition of religious medicine was in contrast to the rational medicine of Hippocrates. The latter sought to account for disease in the natural world. In the former, the source of disease was supernatural. Keep this distinction in mind. As we progress through this book, the conflict between natural and supernatural explanations of phenomena in medicine and elsewhere will arise with great regularity. Even today, in the early twenty-first century, it is with us.

No discussion about religion and medicine in Greece is complete without mentioning the work of the great anatomist Galen, who lived in the second century after Christ. Because dissection of human bodies was prohibited in his time, Galen's theories about bodily function and structure were based on his observations of nonhuman animals. But he stated his conclusions about human physiology with such dogmatism that his views lasted for many centuries, until they were superseded by the work of William Harvey in the seventeenth century. From Galen's perspective, the anatomy he studied demonstrated the perfection of divine design. This view became part of the teachings of Christianity many centuries later.

## MEDICINE IN ROME

Like polytheistic Greece, Rome had no specific gods of healing. A great many gods were responsible for health and illness. Early in the Roman Empire, disease was the result of offending a god. Treatment involved appeasing these gods.

By the mid-second century B.C., Rome had conquered much of the Greek world, absorbing much of its art, architecture, and medicine. The latter included the Greek god Asclepius but also the medicine of Hippocrates; and around 200 B.C., rational medicine began to appear in Rome, largely as a result of the influx of Greek physicians. After initial resistance, to some degree the result of the unpopular practices of the Greek physician Archagathus, who emphasized surgery and cauterization, Greek rational medicine became popular in Rome. As we will soon see, this state of affairs characterizes contemporary America, although not to the same degree.

As the Roman Empire expanded, it absorbed the cultures of the societies it captured. Some of these cultures continued to hold supernatural views about disease, regarding it as demonic possession requiring purification. Others practiced astrology and magic. These beliefs existed alongside the Greek rational medicine that had become accepted in Rome.

## CHRISTIANITY

In Christianity, illness is understood in the context of suffering and redemption. Suffering is essential to the Christian view of the world, and it leads to spiritual renewal. This formulation suggests an inevitable tension between the fate of the soul and the fate of the body. The former is the province of theology; the latter, of medicine. Illness may lead to spiritual growth, and therefore one thread of belief in Christianity has been that illness represents a lack of faith and should not be treated medically. But a somewhat contradictory view has also characterized Christianity. Throughout most of its history, care for suffering and disease by a physician has been viewed not only as acceptable but as a calling, since the physician is an instrument of God.

This latter position is consistent with the practice, beginning in the fourth century, of monastic clergy establishing hospitals along with facilities for the poor and aged. A consistent theme in Christianity is to promote direct ministry to the suffering, providing comfort. This approach encouraged hands-on, practical treatment of disease.

At the same time, however, and in apparent contradiction to this position of providing practical relief to the suffering, accounts of miraculous healing began to increase substantially. Many of these miracles occurred with the use of relics representing saints and martyrs. Thus, in early Christian times, as in most other eras, the relationship between religion, medicine, and magic was a close one. And it existed alongside the impulse toward a more practical medicine that delivered actual care and comfort to the suffering.

In the Middle Ages, after Christianity was well established, belief in the miraculous continued to thrive but so did practical medical care, largely delivered by the clergy. Monasteries continued to provide refuge to the sick and the persecuted. Priests and monks wrote medical treatises. By the late Middle Ages, the Church was involved in granting permission for individuals to practice medicine, as it granted the rights to other professional activities.

In short, until the Renaissance, religion, medicine, and the supernatural overlapped to a considerable degree. For the ancient Egyptians and the Greeks, disease was the result at least in part of the actions of the gods, who expressed their displeasure with human conduct by making people sick. Treatment often involved appeasing these gods. In monotheistic Judaism and Christianity, the connection between appeals to the divine and treatment was less direct, but both religions believe in a connection. For Judaism, faithfulness to God led to a life of health and prosperity. In Christianity, the connection to God was expressed in the view that suffering in this world would lead to divine rewards in the next one.

## THE RISE OF RATIONAL MEDICINE

The intimate link between religion and medicine began to erode during the Renaissance, a separation that was the result of a great many factors. Beginning in the fourteenth century, Europe experienced an intellectual explosion, due in no small part to the rapid development of cities and commercialism not seen in the Middle Ages. One product of this intellectual burst was a challenge to the authority of the Church, the most famous of which was by Martin Luther. The challenge expressed itself more generally in the questioning of Church authority as the primary source of information and in a turn to direct observation.

Observation as a means of acquiring information played a central role in the development of modern medicine and modern science more generally. A primary beneficiary of this new approach was the discipline of anatomy. Renaissance artists expressed a fascination for the human body, producing superb and accurate illustrations. The most famous of these Renaissance artists was Leonardo da Vinci, who produced hundreds of anatomical drawings of startling beauty and accuracy.

But artists were not the only people who had become interested in anatomy. Medical "specialists" also were active, conducting explorations of the structure of the human body in unprecedented ways. Recall that the anatomy of the Greeks and the Romans depended upon dissection of nonhuman animals because dissection of human bodies was prohibited. The literal meaning of the word *autopsy*, "to see with one's own eyes," suggests the role of observation rather than authority in understanding the workings of the body. The anatomists of the Renaissance challenged Galen's physiology by actually observing the structure of *human* bodies.

The fifteenth-century development of the printing press meant that the observations of these anatomists could be published and disseminated widely. One of the greatest of such publications, *De Humani Corporis Fabrica,* written by Vesalius and published in 1543, was a landmark event in anatomy. The *Fabrica* and other similar texts made it clear that observation was the only means by which one could legitimately study the human body.

Reliance on observation instead of authority also influenced the development of the medical disciplines of surgery and therapeutics, although their successes were far more limited than those of anatomy. Indeed, science in general, not just medicine, was transformed by abandoning authority as a source of wisdom and relying instead on the power of observation. The work of Vesalius is a case in point. Initially, he set out to confirm the anatomy of Galen, the authority on this topic for a millennium. But Vesalius discovered mistakes that Galen had made, based largely on the fact that in Galen's time, dissection of the human body was prohibited. Not so in the time of Vesalius. Regrettably for Vesalius, his work was never fully accepted in his lifetime.

The year 1543, when the *Fabrica* was published, was significant not only for medicine but for science in general. It was in that same year that Copernicus published his revolutionary work describing the heliocentric view of the solar system. The significance of this discovery cannot be overemphasized. The idea that the Earth revolved around the Sun and not the other way around fundamentally contradicted the Church's view of the centrality of human existence in the universe. Copernicus's discovery represents a turning point in the history of science, when the method of observation began to overcome the authority of the Church.

All science, medical and otherwise, was on an irrevocable path toward modern empiricism: observation as the method of acquiring knowledge had attained supremacy. Over the next several centuries, science and medicine, freed of the strictures of the Church, developed rapidly. Perhaps the best early example of this new reliance on observation as the primary source of information about the human body is the 1628 discovery of the circulation of the blood by William Harvey in England.

To understand the impact of Harvey's discovery, consider the understanding of the problem he faced. Thirteen hundred years earlier, Galen had theorized that there were different kinds of blood that traveled in different vessels. Nutritive blood was created in the liver and traveled via the veins to all parts of the body, where it was consumed. Some of this nutritive blood, however, went through the vena cava to the heart, where it was infused with vital spirits. According to his theory, the nutritive blood entered the right side of the heart and then crossed to the left side through pores in the septum, the tissue separating the right and left sides of the heart. This "vital blood" then traveled through the arteries, carrying the vital spirits throughout the body. Vital blood reached the brain but not before it was further infused with an animal spirit. When it reached the organs, this animal spirit gave life.

Thus, Galen proposed two different systems of blood connected to each other in the heart. Harvey's dissections demonstrated that Galen's view was wrong in several respects. First, he showed that there were no perforations in the ventricular septum, i.e., that there was no way for blood to move from the right ventricle directly to the left. He also showed that the ventricles contracted together, i.e., expelled blood at the same time. If blood were moving from one ventricle to the other, as Galen had proposed, then one ventricle would be contracting to expel blood while the other relaxed to receive it.

Galen's theory also held that the body's organs consumed blood, which was replenished by the food a person ate. Harvey's evidence demolished this view, too. Again aided by the fact that he could dissect human cadavers, Harvey calculated how much blood the human heart could contain, which would be expelled during each cardiac contraction. Knowing what the average heart rate was, Harvey calculated how much blood passed through the heart in thirty minutes. This amount was so substantial, Harvey reasoned, that it could not possibly be replenished by the food that a person had eaten. Therefore, the blood was not consumed by bodily organs; instead, it must be circulating throughout the body. The heart, Harvey demonstrated, is a pump that is responsible for this circulation. Blood is expelled from the heart to the arterial system and returns to the heart from the veins. This implies quite directly that there must be some other part of the circulatory system that connects the arteries to the veins. Thus, Harvey postulated the existence of the capillary system before Malpighi discovered it in 1661.

This last aspect of Harvey's work provides a perfect illustration of how modern science operates. Harvey had demonstrated that the blood circulated throughout the body, powered by the pumping action of the heart. He further demonstrated that the blood was expelled from the heart into the arterial system and returned to the heart in the venous system. If the blood circulated throughout the body, then the arterial and venous systems must be connected in some way. The technology of the time didn't permit Harvey to discover this connection—the capillaries—but his theory clearly predicted its existence. When a new technology, the microscope, emerged, its use confirmed that capillaries were the connection between the arteries and the veins.

This account nicely illustrates two central features of Harvey's discovery of the circulation of blood. One is the complete absence of references to the supernatural. Harvey believed we could account for bodily phenomena completely without invoking gods or demons or spirits. The second is his thorough reliance on observation and deduction to develop his theory.

For many historians of science, the crowning achievement of the seventeenth century was the 1687 publication of Newton's *Principia,* his masterwork that presented his celestial mechanics, describing the movements of the planets and stars as well as objects here on Earth. This accomplishment was enormous and enduring. More than three hundred years later, the laws Newton described still govern the behavior of the physical phenomena we experience in our everyday lives. Newtonian physics has been supplanted only at the subatomic level.

The *Principia* was not directly relevant to connections between religion, magic, and medicine. But its impact was felt nonetheless because it demonstrated that the laws of physics and mathematics completely explained the physical world. No reference to supernatural forces was required. The discoveries of the anatomists of the seventeenth century made it clear that the body was composed of physical structures whose function could be explained by physical principles without reference to the supernatural. Indeed, the full title of the *Principia* was *Philosophiae Naturalis Principia Mathematica,* the "Mathematical Principles of Natural Philosophy." Medicine from the seventeenth century to the present day has depended almost exclusively on explanations based on natural, as opposed to supernatural, phenomena. Religion had begun to recede as an explanatory principle in medicine.

But as we will see in the next chapter, a movement in the opposite direction has been growing since the latter part of the twentieth century. It threatens the very basis of our modern technological society. The alliance of religion and medicine is an intimate part of this movement.

# 3

FROM *SPUTNIK* TO ANGELS: SCIENCE, SUBJECTIVITY,
AND THE RISE OF IRRATIONALISM

**It's a long way from the seventeenth century to the** mid-twentieth century, and the history of the scientific and medical accomplishments of those years could fill entire libraries. While these achievements were enormous, they were largely the products of the application of the principles and methods that emerged in the sixteenth and seventeenth centuries: an emphasis on observation and experimentation and the diminished influence of authority, whether religious or otherwise, in the search for knowledge. The great discoveries of physics, chemistry, biology, and astronomy in this period were the product of this new and exceptionally fruitful approach that emphasized the centrality of explanations based on the natural, as opposed to the supernatural, world.

Of course, there were exceptions to this trajectory. From the seventeenth to the nineteenth century, a position called *vitalism* held that life was characterized by a vital principle that could not be explained by the laws of the physical world. As a recent op-ed article in *The Washington Post* reported, many geography textbooks of the nineteenth century relied on supernatural explanations of the Earth and the solar system. Neither of these views is held in high esteem today, although descendants of each still exist.

Periodic eruptions of supernaturalism in society have appeared throughout recent history. We are in one such period now, and the evidence is everywhere we look. Popular television programs feature psychic detectives, abductions by aliens, and communication with the dead. Bookstores are filled with self-help books that offer advice on angelic medicine and quantum healing. Modern science is under attack by religious conservatives who prefer biblical accounts of natural phenomena. Given the course of history we just reviewed, how did this happen?

## THE 1950S, THE SOVIET UNION, AND THE COLD WAR

The cold war provides a context for understanding the course of American science in the second half of the twentieth century. Dating roughly from 1945 until 1991, the cold war represented a struggle for global supremacy between the world's two superpowers, the United States and the Soviet Union, distinguished by their economic systems, capitalism and communism respectively. In a book devoted to examining religion and health, we can only superficially address the intellectual context that characterized the 1950s, but even such a limited treatment can provide a framework that makes sense of the rapid rise in interest and support for science during the 1950s.

This decade was characterized by an intense competition between the U.S. and the Soviet Union. The U.S. exploded two atomic bombs in Japan in August 1945. Four years later almost to the day, the Soviet Union successfully tested its own atom bomb. On November 1, 1952, the U.S. exploded the world's first hydrogen bomb. Less than a year later, on August 12, 1953, the USSR duplicated this feat. It was clear that in atomic weapons technology, the race for supremacy was on, and the Soviets were catching up.

This atomic brinksmanship took place with the Korean War as a backdrop. The war began on June 25, 1950, and ended on July 27, 1953. Although it was a conflict between North and South Korea, it generally is regarded as a proxy war between the United States on one side and the Soviet Union and the People's Republic of China on the other. Historians disagree about the number of deaths during the Korean War, but it is safe to say that tens of thousands of U.S. soldiers died. The numbers were far greater for the Koreans and the Chinese. Adding to this stew of low-level terror was the rise, and eventual fall, of Wisconsin's junior senator, Joseph McCarthy, who came to power as a virulent anti-Communist, conducting a campaign of fear and intimidation based on his investigations of government officials and private citizens he accused of being Communists.

Fear of communism and the Soviet Union was widespread in the U.S. and was exacerbated by the Soviets. On October 23, 1956, an uprising against Soviet domination occurred in Hungary, escalating into a full-scale revolt. On November 4 of that year, two hundred thousand Soviet troops and over two thousand tanks entered Hungary, crushing the rebellion. Later that month, Soviet premier Nikita Khrushchev warned Western diplomats, "We will bury you."

## THE SHOCK OF *SPUTNIK*

Into this era of fear came a small metal sphere that crystallized American concerns about the Soviet threat. Shortly after three P.M. eastern time on October 4, 1957, a Soviet intercontinental ballistic missile lifted off from the Baikonur Cosmodrome. It carried a 184-pound, twenty-three-inch-diameter sphere called *Sputnik*. Less than one hour later, *Sputnik,* the first "moon" made by humans, was in Earth's orbit.

By today's standards, the satellite was primitive. All it could do was emit meaningless radio beeps. But it could be seen by the naked eye, and the beeps could be heard by shortwave radio receivers. As the news of the Soviet accomplishment spread, people around the world scrambled to catch a glimpse of the space probe. They climbed onto rooftops and went into their backyards, or into parks if they lived in cities.

Most Americans today were not born when *Sputnik* was launched, so its impact on the country may not be apparent. Set in the context of the cold war competition between the U.S. and the Soviet Union, the successful launch of *Sputnik* had a profound effect on the U.S. Prior to *Sputnik,* it was universally held in America that we were superior to the USSR. That superiority was seen across the board, in culture, in religion, in economics, and in science. And of course that superiority was believed to be due to our free-enterprise system. *Sputnik* put an end to that smug sense of superiority. In fact, it caused a profound anxiety: if the Soviets had the technological capacity to launch a space probe that orbited the Earth, they could attack us from space. Today, we can understand that anxiety in a very real way. As Paul Dickson, author of *"Sputnik": The Shock of the Century,* has put it, the impact of *Sputnik* was similar to the impact we felt after witnessing the events of 9/11.

Certainly, the media perceived how grave the threat was. According to the *Chicago Daily News,* if the Soviets "could deliver a 184-pound 'moon' into a predetermined pattern 560 miles out into space, the day is not far distant when they could deliver a death-dealing warhead onto a predetermined target almost anywhere on the earth's surface." *Newsweek* magazine speculated that *Sputnik*s armed with nuclear weapons could "spew their lethal fallout over the U.S. and Europe." In this sense, the comparison of *Sputnik* to 9/11 is quite apt: both events threatened the perceived invulnerability of the U.S. to attack.

Then-senator Lyndon Johnson's aide George Reedy declared "the simple fact is that we can no longer consider the Russians to be behind us in technology. It took them four years to catch up to our atomic bomb and nine months to catch up to our hydrogen bomb. Now we are trying to catch up to their satellite." Two weeks after *Sputnik,* Nobel Prize–winning physicist I. I. Rabi, who was the chair of President Eisenhower's Scientific Advisory Committee, warned that the Soviet emphasis on education in science and math would put them ahead of us.

But even as the country was reacting with alarm to the success of *Sputnik,* the shock was compounded by the launch of *Sputnik 2.* This satellite was over five times heavier and, more important, it carried a dog. *Sputnik 2* remained in Earth orbit for almost two hundred days.

The magnitude of this technological accomplishment can be understood by the weight of the Soviet space probes. By comparison, the weight of the first American satellite was to be 3.5 pounds.

America had good reason to be concerned about the sudden recognition of the Soviet superiority in science and engineering. On December 6, 1957, the U.S. attempted to match the Soviets in the new space race. The Vanguard rocket carrying satellite TV-3 rose about three feet above the launch pad and then exploded in a fireball. It was an embarrassment of colossal proportions. Unfortunately, the U.S. space program was plagued by many other early and memorable failures. The February 1958 launch of another Vanguard rocket, carrying satellite TV-3BU, also ended in failure. After reaching an altitude of four miles, it exploded. Along with several aborted missions using another rocket, the Jupiter, these failures had the effect of raising questions about whether we would ever match the Soviets. On January 31, 1958, the U.S. succeeded at putting a space probe, *Explorer 1,* into orbit. But it weighed only thirty-one pounds, confirming that the Soviets had much more powerful rockets capable of launching much larger (and potentially lethal) payloads.

## RESPONDING TO *SPUTNIK,* THE U.S. INVESTS IN SCIENCE EDUCATION

In January 1958, Mutual Broadcasting's Gabriel Heatter spoke directly to *Sputnik* in a radio editorial and said, "You suddenly made us realize that we are not the best in everything. You reminded us of an old-fashioned American word, humility. You woke us up out of a long sleep. You made us realize a nation can talk too much, too long, too hard about money. A nation, like a man, can grow soft and complacent. It can fall behind when it thinks it is Number One in everything." Heatter was not alone in his concern.

The cover of the November 18, 1957, issue of *Time* magazine featured physicist Edward Teller, and the cover story was entitled "Knowledge Is Power." Addressing the post-*Sputnik* concern about Soviet superiority in space technology, it reported that the Soviet Union produced more than twice as many scientists and engineers per year as the U.S. In 1957, the article lamented, the U.S. invested about $450 million in basic scientific research, only about 0.1 percent of the gross domestic product. Most staggering was the comparison between the Russian and American educational systems. According to the article, only about 4 percent of American high school students took a course in physics, and only 25 percent took courses in algebra. In the Soviet Union, in contrast, bright students were placed in special schools associated with universities. They took extensive coursework in mathematics, physics, and chemistry. Starting as early as the fourth grade, they studied general science.

In response to this crisis provoked by *Sputnik*, Congress passed the National Defense Education Act (NDEA) in 1958. Historically, education had been regarded as the concern of the states and local communities. In the wake of *Sputnik*, this view was abandoned because of the urgent need to catch up to the Soviets in science and engineering. The federal government would fund education, and the NDEA would promote training in science, math, and foreign languages among other areas. It supported student loans, scholarships, and fellowships, and provided funds for schools to purchase scientific equipment.

In addition, the federal government increased support for the National Science Foundation (NSF). In 1958, the government created two new agencies in response to *Sputnik:* the Advanced Research Projects Agency and the National Aeronautics and Space Administration (NASA).

It wasn't only the physical sciences that benefited from the increased federal aid. Biology, too, was a beneficiary. Evolutionary theory, which had not been taught with much enthusiasm prior to *Sputnik,* was suddenly introduced into the curriculum. *Sputnik* led to an overhaul of American science education in general, not just in the physical sciences.

## THE IMPACT OF THE FEDERAL INVESTMENT

There are many ways to evaluate the impact of the investment of federal funds in scientific research following *Sputnik.* One way, admittedly relatively crude, is to compare the number of American winners of the Nobel Prizes in physics, chemistry, and medicine prior to 1950 and from 1995 to 2005. From 1935 to 1950, American won 3.5 Nobel Prizes in physics, 2 in chemistry, and 4 in medicine. (The fractional prizes reflect the fact that in many years, the Nobel Committee awards a prize to more than a single scientist.) In the ten-year period beginning in 1995, Americans won 7.67 prizes in physics, 5.67 prizes in chemistry, and 6.67 prizes in medicine. Since the Nobel Prizes are awarded years after the prize-winning work is published, this increase in recent years undoubtedly reflects the increased federal investment in science following the shock of *Sputnik.*

Other evidence also demonstrates the impact of the post-*Sputnik* efforts to enhance the role of science in the U.S. As the figure clearly indicates, there was a rapid rise in federal research and development funding beginning in 1958. This sharp increase continued until the mid-1960s, when funding began to fall and then leveled off. Even after leveling off, it was dramatically higher than prior to *Sputnik.*

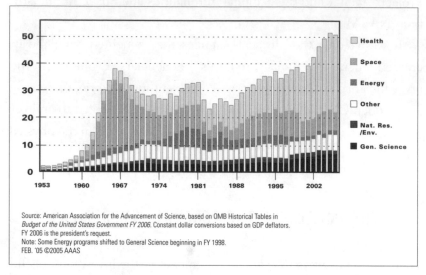

TRENDS IN NONDEFENSE R&D BY FUNCTION, FY 1953–2006
Outlays for the conduct of R&D, billions of constant FY 2005 dollars

Health
Space
Energy
Other
Nat. Res. /Env.
Gen. Science

Source: American Association for the Advancement of Science, based on OMB Historical Tables in *Budget of the United States Government FY 2006*. Constant dollar conversions based on GDP deflators.
FY 2006 is the president's request.
Note: Some Energy programs shifted to General Science beginning in FY 1998.
FEB. '05 ©2005 AAAS

# WHAT SCIENCE IS, AND ISN'T

So it is abundantly clear that in response to the impact of *Sputnik* and the perception of Soviet superiority in the space race, the U.S. began a major increase in the support of science at many different levels. But what, precisely, was being supported? What *is* science and how does it work? To make sense of this history and the current interest in religion and health, we need to answer these questions. We need to understand what science is and what it isn't. In describing the methods of William Harvey, we had a taste of how modern science operates. Now we consider it in greater detail.

## How Science Works

Simply put, science is an organized, systematic approach to acquiring knowledge about natural phenomena. A central and unwavering characteristic is that knowledge is sought by accumulating evidence. Nothing is accepted solely on the basis of faith or authority or personal experience. Correspondingly, scientific theories are constantly evolving, based on the perpetual accumulation of new evidence, which is aggressively pursued. As we'll see later, this description of science contains the seeds of the discontent that, in the late twentieth century, grew into the renewed interest in connections between religion and health.

## Scientific Knowledge Is Based on the Accumulation of Evidence

A central feature of science is that statements are considered true or false based on the accumulation of evidence. Scientists construct hypotheses that can be tested. When hypotheses are not supported by the facts, they are discarded in favor of others more consistent with the facts. Since the time of Galileo in the seventeenth century, all modern science—physics, chemistry, biology, engineering, astronomy, psychology—has operated in this manner. Because of this, we no longer believe in some propositions that at one time were widely held: that the Earth is flat, that the Sun revolves around the Earth, that heavier objects fall faster than lighter ones, or that there are two separate systems of blood circulation.

The heart of this first feature is that science cannot rely on mere authoritative assertions about how things work. After all, the view that the Sun revolved around the Earth was the official position of the Church authorities of the sixteenth century, as well as being consistent with everyday experience. But scientific knowledge cannot depend upon either of these. Nor can it rely on popular opinion or personal beliefs, however heartfelt they may be. Scientific knowledge requires accumulation of evidence that can be observed, replicated, and evaluated by all. Hypotheses that cannot be tested to determine their validity are not scientific. If a hypothesis cannot be proven false, it is not a scientific hypothesis.

This is precisely the reasoning that the courts have followed in determining that "creation science" and "intelligent design" may not be taught in publicly supported science courses. In 1982, a federal district court ruled against an Arkansas law requiring that equal time for the biblical account of creation be provided in science classes that taught Darwinian evolution. The court ruled that creation science is not science precisely because it depends entirely on supernatural intervention and therefore cannot be tested or falsified. In December 2005, Judge John Jones of the U.S. Federal District Court for the Middle District of Pennsylvania came to precisely the same conclusion about intelligent design, the intellectual heir of creationism. Hypotheses that cannot be tested cannot be disproved, and hypotheses that cannot be disproved are not scientific hypotheses.

## Scientific Knowledge Requires Systematic Observation

A second and related characteristic of scientific inquiry is that observations are *systematic;* that is, they are collected in a way that ensures that they are representative of the phenomenon in question. Anecdotal accounts of events, unless accompanied by similar systematic observations, may be highly misleading. The fact that your father-in-law smoked two packs of cigarettes a day for his entire life and still lived to be eighty-five years of age may be a compelling anecdote, but it is not scientific evidence, because it represents only a single case. We can't claim that smoking poses no risk to health unless we look at *many* smokers, not just one. If we look *systematically* at a large sample of smokers and compare them to an equally large sample of nonsmokers, we will see that although there are exceptions, on average the smokers will have shorter lives and will be sicker than the nonsmokers.

## Scientific Knowledge Is Free of Bias

Bias in the scientific sense refers, not to prejudice but rather to threats to the validity of scientific judgments. As philosopher Daniel Dennett has put it, "Scientists take themselves to be just as weak and fallible as anybody else, but recognizing those very sources of error in themselves . . . they devised elaborate systems to tie their own hands, forcibly preventing their frailties and prejudices from infecting their results."

Like the biases associated with prejudice, scientific biases may operate unconsciously and so cloud our judgment. Each individual scientific discipline has its own set of procedures to control bias. Let's examine how the biomedical sciences attempt to avoid bias.

## The Importance of a Control Group

Consider the hypothetical case of a new treatment for headaches. To test this new treatment, a scientist will have to assemble a sample of people with headaches. Their level of pain will be measured and then they will receive the test treatment. Later, the scientist will measure each participant's level of pain again. If the pain after the treatment is lower than before, then we can conclude that the treatment has been effective. Right?

Wrong. In this experimental design, we have not considered the possibility that headaches often disappear on their own. After all, we've all had headaches that got better without intervention. In medicine, this is referred to as *spontaneous remission*. How can we control for the possibility that it might not be the treatment that is responsible for the reduction in pain but rather that the pain has spontaneously remitted?

The simplest way to do this is to take headache sufferers and divide them into two groups: one group will receive the real test treatment medication, and the other will receive a placebo. If we now determine that the active-treatment group experiences greater pain relief than the control group, we are on solid ground in concluding that it was the new treatment and not spontaneous remission that was responsible for the pain reduction. By adding the control group, we have controlled for the bias associated with spontaneous remission.

## The Importance of Sampling from the Entire Population

An essential characteristic of the hypothetical experiment above is that the research subjects be assigned *at random* to the treatment and the control condition. Random assignment was first used as a research tool in 1935 in studies of agricultural productivity. The first biomedical research trial to use it was in 1946, in a study sponsored by the Medical Research Council of England to test the effect of streptomycin on tuberculosis.

Random assignment ensures that there will be no characteristics of individual subjects that might interact with an element of the experiment to skew the findings. In our hypothetical study of the treatment of headache pain, if we didn't assign subjects randomly but let them choose for themselves which treatment condition to be in, then subjects who have a greater sensitivity to pain might be more likely to assign themselves to the active-medication condition than those who were less sensitive to pain. Therefore, if we found that the experimental treatment seemed to produce a greater effect than the placebo, we would not be certain whether this effect was really due to the treatment or to this difference in pain sensitivity among subjects.

The importance of randomization is that we can assume that if we have enough subjects, then all the personal characteristics of subjects that might in some way influence the experimental outcomes will *randomize out,* i.e., they will appear with equal frequency in both the experimental-treatment and placebo conditions. Random assignment assures us that the treatment and control conditions will be identical in all respects *except* in their exposure to the treatment itself. Therefore, if the groups differ in their pain relief, the difference can be attributed only to the treatment and not to some other factor.

## The Importance of the Size of the Sample

In the above experiment on headache pain, we wouldn't be convinced of the superiority of the treatment over the placebo if we had only a single subject in each group. The aim of an experiment is to ensure that the experimental groups are identical to each other in all respects except for the treatment variable. This is accomplished, as we saw above, by randomly assigning subjects to the two groups. But randomization ensures equivalence of groups only if the groups are large enough. We can easily imagine that with a small number of subjects, one group might have more men than women, older subjects than younger ones, healthier subjects than sicker ones. These differences could affect the impact of the treatment; for example, because some evidence suggests that women are more sensitive to pain than men, a group that had more women might have a different response to the treatment than a group having fewer women.

Biomedical scientists have procedures for determining the number of subjects required in a study. These procedures take into consideration the predicted magnitude of the treatment effect and how consistent, or alternatively, how variable, it is. For our purposes, it is unnecessary to go into the details of these procedures, but you should know that they exist. If you're interested, the classic work on this matter is by Jacob Cohen, one of the great figures in statistics.

## The Rosenthal Effect: How a Researcher's Expectations Can Affect the Outcome of an Experiment

One well-established bias in conducting scientific research is that an experimenter's expectations can subtly but substantially influence the outcome of that inquiry. The classic case of this bias is called the Rosenthal effect, named after Harvard psychologist Robert Rosenthal, who conducted many of the studies that identified this phenomenon. It has also been called the *expectancy effect* or the *self-fulfilling prophecy*. In addition to threatening the validity of scientific research, it has substantial implications for our everyday lives.

One classic study by Rosenthal used laboratory animals to demonstrate the expectancy effect. Rats can learn to negotiate a maze if they receive reinforcement for their efforts. In a typical learning study, a hungry rat will be placed at the beginning of the maze, and after wandering aimlessly through it for some time, it will, quite by accident, find its way to the end, where it will receive food reinforcement. The study proceeds by additional trials in the maze, with each successful effort by the rat resulting in reinforcement. Over time, the rat will learn the maze and will be able to run directly from the start box to the finish making no wrong turns. Early trials are characterized by many wrong turns and long times to run from the start box to the finish. But as the trials progress, the rats make fewer and fewer mistakes and correspondingly reach the finish faster and faster.

Rosenthal and colleagues led student experimenters conducting such learning studies to believe that they were working with rats that had been specially bred either to excel at learning to negotiate mazes or to be poor at maze performance. These students then conducted the maze studies as described above. As Rosenthal predicted, the "maze bright" rats performed better than the "maze dull" rats: they learned to run from the start box to the finish more quickly.

The problem was that in fact there was no difference between the "maze bright" and "maze dull" rats. They were selected randomly from the same large colony. The difference in performance was due, not to characteristics of the rats but rather to the expectations of the students who conducted the experiments. Those expectations led the students with the "bright" rats to be more satisfied with the study. They were more friendly toward their rat subjects and were more relaxed with them. That is, they appeared to treat them better than the students with the "dull" rats.

Rosenthal reasoned that the same effect of expectations could influence the performance of schoolchildren. To test this hypothesis, students were administered an intelligence test at the beginning of the school year. Teachers were told that this test would predict intellectual blooming; children scoring high on this test were expected to show substantial intellectual gains during the school year. *The teachers were told which students were expected to bloom.*

At the end of the school year, all the children were tested again, and those students identified as intellectual bloomers performed significantly better in this second test than the other students. As in the study with the laboratory rats, there were in fact no differences between the children. The only difference was in the expectations that the teachers had of them, and these expectations led to superior performance. We can surmise that, just as in the rat study, the "bright" students were subtly treated better by their teachers than the "dull" ones.

It's not hard to imagine how this could happen. A question by a "bright" student would be interpreted by the teacher as showing intellectual curiosity, whereas the same question by a dull student would indicate how limited this student really was. Teachers would be more likely to pay attention to the "bright" students than the "dull" ones. Over the course of a year, these subtle but real differences would have an impact on the students, so that by the end of the year, the "bright" students really would perform better on the intelligence test than the "dull" ones. The expectations truly would become self-fulfilling.

Both the animal and the human studies show the powerful effect of expectations on outcomes in research studies. The point of these studies is obvious: the expectations that researchers and subjects have about the outcome of the studies they conduct can heavily bias those outcomes. The obvious way to eliminate this bias is to require that both the researchers and the subjects be *blind* to the experimental conditions; that is, neither the researchers nor the subjects can know which experimental condition they are assigned to. In a *double-blind* study of the effect of a treatment, neither the researchers nor the subjects will know which subjects receive the real treatment and which ones receive only the placebo.

Double-blind studies are easy to conduct in experiments to test the efficacy of new medicines, where we can control which subjects will receive the active treatment and which will receive the placebo. Currently at Columbia University, we are conducting one such study, to test the impact of a drug on depression resulting from a medical condition. We don't know whether our research subjects receive the active medication or the placebo, and neither do they. Only the research pharmacy, which bottled the medicines, knows the difference. After the study is over, we will "break the blind" and analyze the data. But in the meantime, neither we nor the subjects will have expectations that could influence the outcomes, because no one knows who receives the active medication and who receives the placebo.

Unfortunately, to answer many important questions in medicine, we lack this kind of experimental control. That is, there are many instances in biomedical science in which we cannot conduct an experiment that allows us to randomly assign subjects to a treatment or control group and to conceal from both the scientists and the subjects who receives the real treatment and who receives only the placebo.

## How a Scientist Conducts Research When Total Control Is Impossible

All scientific inquiry attempts to eliminate bias in drawing causal inferences. The experiment, in which a scientist has the capacity to control all the factors that can influence the outcome in question, is ideally designed to accomplish this objective. But there are many areas of science in which conducting experiments is difficult if not impossible. In the field of astronomy, for example, scientists cannot control the phenomena under investigation. An astronomer cannot make star A move in a certain way to determine its effect on planet B. Similarly in the earth sciences, scientists cannot control the geological forces that led to the creation of the Grand Canyon. Therefore, in sciences like astronomy and the earth sciences, experiments are impossible, and scientists must resort to other methods of inquiry.

In the biomedical and psychosocial sciences, too, conducting experiments is frequently impossible. For example, a substantial body of evidence demonstrates that depression is associated with heart disease. Ideally, from a purely scientific perspective, we would conduct an experiment in which we would randomly make some subjects depressed and others not depressed and then follow them for years, after which we would test them for heart disease. If, in this hypothetical experiment, the depressed group developed more heart disease than the nondepressed group, we would be justified in concluding that depression caused heart disease.

But, as the hypothetical nature of this experiment demonstrates, this is impossible. We cannot take a group of volunteer subjects and, by random assignment, make half of them depressed and half not depressed and then follow them. Even if we could make them depressed, it would be highly unethical. Nor can we make people schizophrenic or not, give them enriched or deprived upbringings, higher or lower IQs, black or white skin, high or low income, male or female gender, or religious or nonreligious orientations. Under these conditions, conducting an experiment to determine the effect of gender, race, IQ, socioeconomic status, or religious status on some outcome variable is impossible. We need an alternate research strategy.

## Observational Studies

When we investigate the effects of factors like these, we rely on a different scientific approach to determine their relationships to health outcomes. Because in these cases we have no experimental control over these variables, we are forced to select people who already differ from each other in the characteristics of interest. That is, if we were interested in studying the relationship between income and mortality, we would have to identify and select groups of people with different income levels and then follow them until enough of the sample died to justify drawing conclusions.

So, for example, we might classify all people who earned less than

$50,000 a year as one group and all the others, whose income exceeded $50,000, as the other group. Then we could follow these subjects for years until enough died for us to draw conclusions about the impact of income on mortality.

That would be simple enough to do, but the interpretation of the findings might not be so clear. If we could conduct an experiment and control which subjects had high incomes and which had low incomes, we could unequivocally draw a conclusion about the effect of income on mortality. We could do this because in an experiment, we assure ourselves and others that the *only* difference between the groups is the level of income. That is, no other factor is responsible for the effect.

But we can't conduct such an experiment, so all we can do is *select* people who differ in income level. The problem with this approach is that there are many other factors that go hand in hand with personal income that also might influence the outcome: mortality. For example, we know that the diets of poor and wealthy people differ considerably, with the former receiving poorer nutrition. We know that the wealthy have different jobs than the less well off in the population, that they have access to better housing, better education, better health care, and less physically demanding work, to name a few, all of which also have an effect on mortality.

So the challenge for us is to be able to determine the association between income and mortality after attempting to rule out the effect of these other factors. If we fail to do this, we run the serious risk of drawing biased conclusions. Later, we'll discuss how biomedical researchers deal with this problem.

Right now let's look at the three sources of bias that we covered above. We saw that spontaneous remission, lack of random assignment, and experimenter expectations all had the potential to bias findings in a way that would make them questionable. In an experiment, we could control them by using a control group, randomly assigning subjects to different experimental conditions, and insisting that researchers (and research subjects) be blind to the conditions they were in.

Unfortunately, in observational studies, none of these approaches is possible. In an observational study, we cannot create a control group, i.e., a group that is identical to the experimental group in all respects except that one group receives the active treatment while the other receives a placebo. We can't do this precisely because the variables we are interested in cannot be controlled by the experimenter. So we are left with a situation in which subjects *self-select* which condition they are in. In the case of smoking, some subjects choose to smoke and others choose not to. So not only can we not create a control group to control for the possibility of spontaneous remission, we also cannot randomly assign subjects to different experimental conditions. Finally, because subjects self-select, they are not blind to their assignment. They *know* whether they smoke or not. Similarly, investigators also know this information.

Thus, observational studies are far less able than experimental studies to control the sources of bias that threaten the validity of conclusions we might draw from them. This doesn't mean that we should never conduct observational studies, because if we didn't, we'd be unable to study many important problems. And as we'll see later, there are other methods for addressing some of these threats to valid inferences. But they are not as powerful as those available in experimental studies.

To summarize, the aim of science is to understand how the natural world operates. Biology, chemistry, physics, geology, medicine, psychology, and astronomy, to name a few fields, all follow certain basic principles. They depend upon systematic observation. They employ methods that attempt to identify the connections between events and phenomena in an unbiased way. And they state their hypotheses in ways that allow for testing and, importantly, for disconfirmation. Hypotheses based on supernatural explanations cannot be scientific, because they can never be disconfirmed. Reliance on authority or faith or subjectivity has no place in science.

It is these characteristics that have led to conflicts with the cultural forces that arose in the late twentieth century in the U.S. and paved the way for the rising interest in religion and health.

## CHANGING ATTITUDES TOWARD SCIENCE

In the post-*Sputnik* period, American attitudes toward science were extremely positive, as we might expect. Although these attitudes resulted from the successes the U.S. eventually had in the space program, other factors also contributed. Among the most significant was the development in the mid-1950s of the polio vaccine, the "shot" heard 'round the world. On April 12, 1955, the development of a successful vaccine to prevent polio, an epidemic that had disabled or paralyzed thousands, mostly children, was announced.

A 1981 review of several surveys documented this high regard for science in the post-*Sputnik* period. According to the review, a 1957–58 national opinion poll found that 83 percent of respondents believed that the world was a better place because of science. But in response to similar questions asked of survey respondents in 1972, 1974, and 1976, participants, although still supportive of science, were less so. Only 70 percent, 75 percent, and 71 percent agreed that science made the world a better place. Correspondingly, by 1976 the proportion of respondents who had negative or ambivalent attitudes toward science had doubled, compared to the data from 1957. Georgine Pion and Mark Lipsey, the authors of this review, wrote, "We might conclude that the seeds of disenchantment with science and technology are present."

Other survey data suggest that in the years since this 1981 report, support for science has stabilized at 70 to 75 percent. Although this level of support is still high, it is substantially lower than in the immediate post-*Sputnik* period. And as Pion and Lipsey anticipated, the seeds of disenchantment with science have germinated and grown.

Even if we hold science in high esteem, Americans generally know little about it. Surveys commissioned by the National Science Foundation have asked respondents to explain in their own words how to study something scientifically. The answers suggest that about two-thirds of all Americans do not understand what it means to approach a problem scientifically.

Our knowledge of some scientific facts is greater. More than 70 percent of respondents to this survey knew that oxygen comes from plants and that light travels faster than sound. However, fewer than half knew that it takes the Earth one year to revolve around the Sun and that the earliest humans and dinosaurs did not live at the same time. Questions about the origin of the universe and the evolution of humans were correctly answered by fewer than 50 percent of the respondents, a fact the report attributes to confusion of religious belief and scientific information.

Not surprisingly, recent evidence shows that compared to students in other advanced industrial countries, U.S. students perform poorly in tests of science and mathematics. Scores from the Third International Mathematics and Science Study in 2003 showed that by eighth grade, U.S. students were only in the middle of the distribution of developed countries. By the end of high school, U.S. students were in last place. Intertwined with the decline in favorable attitudes toward science and the emergence of scientific illiteracy in the U.S. is the rise of the ethos of subjectivity.

## THE SELF-HELP MOVEMENT AND SUBJECTIVITY

In her wonderful book *Sleeping with Extra-Terrestrials,* social critic Wendy Kaminer examines the rise in irrationalism in the U.S. during the 1980s and 1990s. She makes the compelling case that the New Age, recovery, self-help, and emerging fundamentalist religious movements of the 1970s through the 1990s contributed heavily to a reverence for subjectivity at the expense of fact. Personal growth and knowledge, Kaminer observes, are, in one way or another, the aim of all of these movements. "All we know is what we perceive, and all that we perceive, or feel, deserves 'validation.'" "The therapeutic culture and related New Age 'consciousness' movements, for example, have already infected the political sphere with a preference for feelings over facts." Pop spirituality, in her view, is nonjudgmental about almost all matters except, of course, rationality. In this new century, the truth often seems based more on sincerity, intensity, and ubiquity of belief than on evidence. This attitude is antithetical to science and is consistent with a growing embrace of the supernatural.

I was surprised to see evidence of this ethos of subjectivity when, just recently, I was interviewed by a very seasoned broadcast journalist for a program he was putting together. Our topic was the press coverage of the religion and health issue. He told me that while preparing for his article on the topic, he had interviewed a great many people who reported to him that their religious activities were responsible for their successful recovery from illness. He was so impressed with the sincerity of their beliefs that despite the fact that he had been in the journalism business for forty years and should have been skeptical of unsubstantiated anecdotal accounts, he nonetheless concluded that there must be something to the claims that religion is good for your health. It's disconcerting that such an experienced journalist would believe this, but it makes Kaminer's point: these days, information is based more on sincerity and subjectivity than evidence.

Rationality, Kaminer writes, is founded on skepticism—skepticism about all beliefs, including one's own. This stance requires that all beliefs be subjected to scrutiny and debate and empirical verification to determine their validity. This, of course, is the basis of science: that beliefs are considered facts only if they are supported by evidence, and evidence is based on objectivity, not subjectivity.

Kaminer's observations were astonishingly prescient. *Sleeping with Extra-Terrestrials* was published in 1999; in the intervening years, we have seen examples of the reverence for subjectivity over rationality virtually every day. "Flights from reason take off in our day as frequently as planes from O'Hare."

This lack of understanding of science and the infatuation with subjectivity are responsible for the enormous popularity of pseudoscience in the U.S. Contemporary science is criticized for being excessively "linear" and "reductionist." Preferable approaches to wisdom are spiritual, holistic, and nonlinear. That is, they don't have to make sense. People appear to be more interested in being guided by angelic voices than by scientific information.

A June 8, 2001, Gallup poll assessed popular opinions about psychic and paranormal phenomena. According to this survey, 54 percent of the respondents believed that psychic or spiritual power could heal the body. This represented an 8 percent increase compared to the results from a 1990 Gallup survey. According to the same 2001 poll, 32 percent of respondents believed in clairvoyance, up 6 percent from 1990, and 28 percent believed that people can communicate with the dead, up 10 percent from 1990.

A February 2002 CBS News poll found that 57 percent of Americans believe in extrasensory perception, telepathy, or other experiences that science cannot explain. Similarly, a Harris poll conducted in February 2003 showed that 84 percent of those surveyed believed in miracles, 51 percent in ghosts, 31 percent in astrology, and 27 percent in reincarnation. Data from a June 16, 2005, Gallup poll show little change from these findings. Overall, 75 percent of those polled believed in at least one of ten common pseudoscientific phenomena, while only 27 percent believed in none at all. Other polling data show similar findings.

Thus, the U.S. is awash in pseudoscientific beliefs—and it's good business, too, if sales of books are any reflection. Bookstores are full of volumes about angels, spirits, fairies, and miracles. In *Angel Medicine*, Dr. Doreen Virtue writes that during a recent trip to the Greek island Santorini, she was contacted by a group of angels from Atlantis who took her on a spiritual adventure, leading her to uncover ancient healing secrets. Fortunately, she discovered that her own personal experience with angelic healing described in many other books (also for sale) was perfectly consistent with the messages of the angels from Atlantis. Apparently, the angels offer all sorts of advice. In *Healing with Fairies,* Dr. Virtue writes that the angels recommended that she reduce her chocolate consumption. Amazon.com has 104 products by Doreen Virtue for sale, but she's small potatoes compared to spirituality guru Deepak Chopra: Amazon has 1,026 products by him.

Many have complained that there is no evidence for angels. Consistent with the reliance on subjectivity and disavowal of rationality, the new age spiritual response to this complaint is that the angels reveal themselves only to those ready to embrace them.

Popular gurus like Chopra, Virtue, Wayne Dyer, and dozens of others sell books and spirituality-related paraphernalia by the millions. Americans, it appears, love to graze at the spiritual buffet, as Wendy Kaminer has put it. These "works" are supplemented by workshops offered around the country and internationally. These workshops promise to transform the lives of participants, but this kind of enlightenment isn't free. A November 2005 "Celebrate Your Life" two-day workshop featuring an all-star cast of New Age gurus like Chopra and Dyer cost between $345 and $470, depending upon how early you registered. If you wanted to purchase preferred seating in the first ten rows (limited availability only), you could do so for $530. And, of course, there were the inevitable pre- and postconference workshops, available to you for additional fees.

More elaborate was the program offered in Assisi, Italy, in April 2006. For $2,599 (including airfare!), you could enjoy five days of intensive workshops led by Alan Cohen and Pat Rodegast. According to the program's Web site, you could "experience Pat Rodegast channeling Emmanuel's gentle, loving and truthful wisdom and Alan Cohen as he teaches you how to make life choices in harmony with your true intentions and live your passion . . . all in the exquisite surroundings as you explore Assisi, Italy!" Apparently, Emmanuel is a spirit who offers the enduring wisdom of the ages. Of course, books, audiotapes, and CDs by these workshop leaders will be available for purchase.

In the past, achieving spiritual enlightenment required conducting an ascetic life. You had to give up material pleasures. Not anymore. Now you can attain enlightenment *and* material wealth, and with relative ease. Alan Cohen offers workshops that will teach you how to "have it all." Wayne Dyer's *Manifest Your Destiny* describes "nine spiritual principles for getting everything you want." In *The Seven Spiritual Laws of Success,* Deepak Chopra tells us how, once we learn our true nature and how to live in harmony with natural law, we will be able to create enormous wealth effortlessly. Spirituality is a means to achieve one's wishes. Books like these are bestsellers.

It is tempting to conclude that these books and workshops are harmless entertainment. After all, no one is forced to purchase them, and they are probably no less socially redeeming than sports or movies. But in fact they represent a corrosive societal influence. By advancing subjectivity at the expense of rationality, they threaten the scientific and technological achievements of our modern society. Industry, medicine, and commerce all are completely indebted to science and technology, and embracing subjectivity as an alternative to rationality will lead to the end of science and the benefits it has brought us. Ironically, the technological advances like mass media and the Internet that permit Deepak Chopra and others to ply their spiritual wares would not be available if we as a society had pursued the antiscience agenda these gurus recommend. There would be no airplanes to fly to international workshops that promise enlightenment.

Much of the support for pursuing connections between religion and health is based on favoring subjectivity over rationality, faith over reason. Because religion relies heavily on faith, it need not depend upon the objectivity that science demands. Religious truths do not require scientific verification. To suggest otherwise is to completely misunderstand the nature of faith. But science, as we have seen, operates according to a different set of rules. For this very reason, religious truths are not scientific ones. The embrace of subjectivity in the late twentieth century has muddied this distinction, helping neither science nor religion. It has, though, contributed to an environment conducive to the linking of religion, spirituality, and health in a dangerous embrace that threatens the progress of contemporary medicine.

# 4

## WHY NOW?

In reviewing this history of religion and medicine, we saw that they, along with magic, have been intertwined for most of human history and only recently were separated, however incompletely. We also saw how with the Enlightenment, medicine began to change fundamentally, abandoning an approach based on authority in favor of one increasingly dependent upon observation. Of course, it wasn't only medicine that was affected by these changes. All of science began to explode when it was freed to explore natural phenomena by controlled and systematic observation.

Since the time of the Enlightenment, science in general and medicine specifically have been dominated by this intellectual tradition of empiricism. The accomplishments of science and medicine are far too numerous to catalog. As we discussed in the previous chapter, social movements of the late twentieth century contributed to a decline in the appreciation of this empirical tradition and a parallel rise in an environment characterized by irrationalism. No doubt these changes have contributed to the emergence of an interest in reconnecting medicine and religion. But for this interest to flourish as it has at the turn of the twenty-first century, other factors had to be involved. There have been at least four such factors worth considering:

- Dissatisfaction with contemporary medicine in the U.S.
- Advocacy foundations and other groups that have leveraged their resources, often considerable, to promote connections between religion and health
- An uncritical media, increasingly driven by market forces, that present stories about religion and health because they are popular with the general public
- Cyclical increases and decreases of religious sentiments that have characterized American society for centuries

In this chapter, we examine each of these factors.

## THE BACKLASH: CONTEMPORARY DISSATISFACTION WITH MODERN MEDICINE

The accomplishments of contemporary medicine as practiced in the U.S. and the rest of the Western world have been extraordinary. Advances in pharmaceuticals, surgery, diagnostic imaging, and public health contributed to an increased life expectancy in the U.S. from forty-nine to seventy-seven years over the course of the twentieth century.

Paralleling this increase in life expectancy are increases in the survival rates for individuals with certain diseases or undergoing certain types of medical treatments. Today, an infant born with cystic fibrosis has an average life expectancy of forty-five years. In 1960, the same infant was expected to live only five years. In 1960, the five-year survival rate for all types of leukemia was about 14 percent. Today it is about 50 percent. At the beginning of the twentieth century, surgery was primitive and often resulted in death. At the beginning of the twenty-first century, surgeons routinely transplant any number of organs and tissues with great success. Surgical procedures that once required long hospitalizations now are performed on an outpatient basis. But recently, despite this progress, dissatisfaction with modern Western medicine has arisen. In August 2005, *The New York Times* ran a devastating series on the experience of being a patient. It presented a sobering account of the pervasive dissatisfaction with the experience of modern medicine in the U.S. Here is an excerpt from this report.

> *Mary Duffy was lying in bed half-asleep on the morning after her breast cancer surgery in February when a group of white-coated strangers filed into her hospital room.*
>
> *Without a word, one of them—a man—leaned over Ms. Duffy, pulled back her blanket, and stripped her nightgown from her shoulders.*
>
> *Weak from the surgery, Ms. Duffy, 55, still managed to exclaim, "Well, good morning," a quiver of sarcasm in her voice.*
>
> *But the doctor ignored her. He talked about carcinomas and circled her bed like a presenter at a lawnmower trade show, while his audience, a half-dozen medical students in their 20's, stared at Ms. Duffy's naked body with detached curiosity, she said.*
>
> *After what seemed an eternity, the doctor abruptly turned to face her.*
>
> *"Have you passed gas yet?" he asked.*
>
> *"Those are his first words to me, in front of everyone," said Ms. Duffy."*

It's hard to find a better example of the insensitivity of contemporary medicine as practiced in the U.S. today. Despite demonstrable improvements in many indices of health—reductions in deaths due to cardiovascular disease, improved treatment of infectious disease, vastly superior surgical procedures—the *experience* of being a patient has worsened. According to a recent survey of more than two thousand adults, 55 percent reported dissatisfaction with the quality of health care, a substantial increase since 2000.

In his annual review of the year for MSNBC, Dr. Arthur Caplan, director of the Center for Bioethics at the University of Pennsylvania, called our health care system the biggest moral failure of 2004. He observed that waiting times in emergency rooms around the country routinely exceed seven hours. Hospital administrators spend long hours arguing with representatives from managed-care organizations about whether patients can receive certain medical treatments and if so, for how long. And, of course, as Caplan reported, the patients in these cases are the fortunate ones because they actually have health insurance. More than 45 million Americans don't. He concluded that in many American hospitals, the level of cleanliness is no better than that found in hospitals in Bangladesh or Bolivia, third world countries whose medical care is thought to be far below that of the U.S.

Here's an illuminating example. A neighbor recently told me of an aborted vacation in England. While visiting there, he suffered a pulmonary embolism, an extremely serious condition in which a blood clot lodges in the lungs. It can lead to a heart attack or stroke. He was treated for eight days in a London hospital. Despite the fact that he was in a ward with many other patients, his experience was extremely satisfying. The nursing staff was courteous and solicitous. Physicians treated him with respect and concern. He felt treated like a person, not a "pulmonary embolism case." He left with an acute awareness of how different the experience of being a patient was in the UK compared to the U.S. This dissatisfaction with the U.S. system is increasingly common, and evidence of it appears everywhere. In the popular 1997 movie *As Good As It Gets,* the daughter of Carol Connelly, played by Helen Hunt, has a chronic illness and receives scandalously insensitive and inadequate medical care. During one visit to the doctor, Ms. Hunt screams, "Goddamn HMOs!"; at a showing of the film, the audience erupted with applause. Clearly, this sentiment struck a responsive chord. We crave more personal, more caring treatment by the health care system. We want to be treated like people, not cases with one disease or another, not collections of tissues and organ systems.

As you might expect, there are many reasons why the experience of being a patient has changed. Attempts to treat medicine like a market commodity have resulted in policies that influence which doctors patients can see and interpose a mountain of paperwork between the treatment the doctors deliver and the payment they may eventually (but do not always) receive. Physicians increasingly are members of "panels" of practitioners created by insurance companies for the purpose of controlling costs. By joining these panels, physicians receive patient referrals, but in exchange, they agree to accept reduced fees for their services. To compensate for these reduced fees, they attempt to see greater numbers of patients, thus reducing the amount of time they spend with any single patient. They also compensate for the reduced income by ordering a greater number of diagnostic tests. Reduced time with the physician and more time spent being tested or discussing the test results contributes to a more impersonal, less satisfying patient experience. The quality of the contact that remains has been thoroughly degraded.

Another element of this managed-care environment in the U.S. today is the oversight requirements imposed by the third-party payers, the insurance companies. Virtually every physician these days complains about being swamped with paperwork required to justify that the treatments they prescribe are necessary. And of course, each insurance company is different in the oversight and corresponding documentation it requires. This burden is also experienced by patients who are understandably mystified by limitations on the treatment their doctors say is necessary.

The medical advances of the twentieth century produced an unprecedented degree of specialization that in turn led to an unintended and unfortunate consequence. For all their power, advances in medical technology have had a dehumanizing effect on the experience of being a patient. MRIs and CT scans, invasive procedures like cardiac catheterization and colonoscopies may have revolutionized diagnostic testing, but the personal experience of these tests leaves a great deal to be desired. The increased reliance on advanced medical technology further erodes the quality of human contact in medicine.

These changes have led us to feel a lack of control over our medical fate. In a less technological era, our interactions with the medical system were on a more human scale, and we could understand some basic elements of our condition and how we were supposed to behave in treating it. Very little of today's medicine is anything like this.

So for many reasons—financial, scientific, technological, political—the experience of being a patient in the U.S. in the early twenty-first century has become dissatisfying, to say the least.

One response to these changes has been the astonishing embrace of complementary and alternative medicine (CAM). In an influential paper published in 1993, Harvard researcher David Eisenberg and colleagues reported that a very substantial fraction of U.S. adults had used at least one of a great many CAM techniques such as chiropractic, massage, imagery, homeopathy, and energy healing, to name a few. More recently, José Pagán and Mark Pauly reported that 61 percent of patients they surveyed had used one of seventeen CAM practices that included prayer, spiritual healing, relaxation techniques, and yoga.

The reasons for this explosion of interest in CAM should be obvious. CAM practices are far less technological and on a more human scale than modern technological medicine and allow patients to experience some sense of control over their medical fates. Providers of CAM offer something that used to be routine in conventional medical care: a human connection between the patient and the physician.

It is in this context that interest in the role of religion in contemporary medicine has grown. Considering religious practices as treatments for disease is in many ways comforting. They are familiar and reassuring. Unlike high-technology medical treatments that are incomprehensible and potentially frightening to patients, religious practices are understandable and comforting. Patients may know at least as much about them as physicians do.

Bringing religion into clinical medicine may be satisfying for both patients and physicians. Engaging in discussions of religious and spiritual matters during clinical visits is experienced by the patient as a valued interpersonal experience, one that is a great relief from discussions about the results of the most recent MRI or blood-chemistry analysis. For physicians, too, conversations about religious and spiritual matters can provide an island of human contact in an otherwise technological sea. Patients aren't the only ones who lament the degradation of the physician-patient relationship.

But neither solution—alternative medicine or religion and medicine—is necessarily a good solution to the problems of dehumanized modern medicine. H. L. Mencken, the "bard of Baltimore," wrote, "For every complex problem, there is a solution that is simple, neat, and wrong." Bringing religious practices into contemporary clinical medicine may be simple and neat, but like treating a symptom instead of the underlying cause, it is misguided and wrong. As we will see in later chapters, the evidence that religious practices affect health is extremely weak. And the mixing of religion and medicine raises substantial ethical, practical, and even theological issues.

The solution to the problem of impersonal medicine is not to abandon the advances made by medical science but to *deliver health care based on those advances in a sensitive, caring way.* Contemporary doctors can treat patients as whole people and in a sensitive manner without embracing approaches that have little scientific support for their effectiveness and for which physicians have little or no training. Of course, this is not a simple matter, given the enormous political and financial obstacles that exist, but pursuing solutions that are simple, neat, and wrong is not the answer.

# THE ROLE OF ADVOCACY ORGANIZATIONS

No single organization has been more responsible for the rising interest in religion and medicine than the John Templeton Foundation. Based in Pennsylvania and endowed by the wealth of financier Sir John Templeton, the foundation's mission, according to its Web site, is "to stimulate a high standard of excellence in scholarly understanding which can serve to encourage further worldwide explorations of the moral and spiritual dimensions of the Universe and of the human potential within its ultimate purpose." The aim of the foundation's initiative on spirituality and health is to document "the positive medical aspects of spiritual practice" and thus "contribute to the reintegration of faith into modern life." Note that the foundation does not propose to explore *whether* there are positive medical aspects of spiritual practice. It assumes that they exist and aims only to document them— risking the dangers of the Rosenthal effect we discussed earlier.

Templeton has provided funding for many of the high-profile researchers in the field. Drs. Harold Koenig, Dale Matthews, David Larson, Jeffrey Levin, Herbert Benson, and Michael McCullough all have been the recipients of Templeton support. Of course, there is nothing wrong with receiving support from foundations for research. Indeed, foundations play an important role in supporting research in biomedicine.

The problem arises when the research supported by foundations is substandard. For most biomedical research, the gold standard is funding by the National Institutes of Health (NIH). To receive funding from the NIH, researchers submit *detailed* proposals about the studies they plan to conduct. These proposals can be well over fifty pages long, sometimes much longer. Proposals are reviewed by groups of other scientists with relevant expertise, and they often decide that proposals are unworthy of funding. These proposals are rejected.

In contrast, proposals to most foundations are typically far shorter and much less detailed, and receive far less scrutiny. Foundation support for biomedical research in the U.S. is critically important, and while some foundations are as selective about recipients as the NIH, most—including those that fund research in religion and health—are not.

Enter the Templeton Foundation. Harold Koenig has been particularly fortunate. Many of his research papers acknowledge support from the Templeton Foundation. Dr. Koenig is the editor of *Science and Theology News,* a Templeton-supported newsletter. The Duke Center for Spirituality, Theology and Health is supported by funds from the Templeton Foundation; Dr. Koenig is the center's director. The Templeton Foundation Press has published two of his books.

But Dr. Koenig is not the only recipient of Templeton support. The foundation spent $2.4 million on the enormous Study of the Therapeutic Effects of Intercessory Prayer, a study of distant intercessory prayer directed by Herbert Benson that will be discussed in Chapter 9. Books by Herbert Benson, Dale Matthews, and Jeffrey Levin acknowledge Templeton support, either directly or through other organizations supported by the foundation.

Thus, the Templeton Foundation has contributed substantially to the publication of research papers suggesting relationships between religious practices and health. We can only speculate what the fate of these papers would have been without that support.

Templeton has also supported promoting a connection between religion and health in other, innovative ways. In 1991, an organization called the National Institute for Healthcare Research (NIHR) was founded in Rockville, Maryland. The NIHR's mission was to "objectively" examine the role that religion and spirituality might play in physical and mental health. Its name and this location were unlikely to be accidental. Rockville is the home of several of the institutes of the NIH. Locating the NIHR in Rockville and calling it the National Institute of Healthcare Research might suggest that this "institute" was part of the federally funded NIH, the foremost biomedical research organization in the world. But the NIHR was not part of the NIH. It was the product of the largesse of the John Templeton Foundation.

According to the Media Transparency Web site, the NIHR received 124 awards totaling $8,025,772 from 1998 to 2002. Every award came from the John Templeton Foundation.

In its heyday, the NIHR was home to some of the most productive contributors to the field, who aimed to demonstrate a connection between religion and health. Their names should be familiar to you by now: Dale Matthews, David Larson, Jeffrey Levin, Michael McCullough, and Christina Puchalski. In the course of its existence, the NIHR convened meetings, funded research studies, and issued "consensus" reports and press releases, all with the aim of demonstrating that religious involvement was good for your health. The NIHR was responsible for any number of mediocre research studies and exaggerated claims about evidence.

Among its most significant products was *The Faith Factor,* a multivolume "systematic" review of the literature on religion and health. The authors of this review were David Larson, James Swyers, and Michael McCullough. Like its successor, the *Handbook of Religion and Health* (which we'll cover in Chapter 7), it was filled with misleading statements and crude and careless analyses.

But if the purpose of the game is to advance the public perception that religion is good for your health, Templeton has been very successful. It has leveraged its support extremely effectively. In addition to providing direct support to individual researchers, Templeton has funded many programs on science, religion, and medicine. Currently, the foundation promotes bringing religion and spirituality into medical education by issuing awards for medical school curricula in religion, spirituality, and medicine, such as the Spirituality and Medicine Curricular Award for Medical Schools and the Spirituality and Medicine Award for Primary Care Residency Training Programs. Through these programs, the foundation attempts to change the way medical education is delivered. Each program aims to promote the involvement of physicians in the religious and spiritual lives of their patients.

*Science and Theology News,* the monthly newsletter supported by

Templeton and edited by Dr. Harold Koenig, claims a readership of thirty thousand. As its name suggests, it covers the relationship between science and religion but also focuses extensively on health. On September 21, 2005, the newsletter's Web site contained a link to the lasting legacy of David Larson. This link presented an interview about Dr. Larson with Dr. Jeffrey Levin. The role of the Templeton Foundation in supporting this religion-and-medicine mutual admiration society could not be clearer.

The Web site also contains a link to a newly published collection of Dr. Larson's writings—edited by Drs. Jeffrey Levin and Harold Koenig. Both the Web site for this book and the book itself contain the following endorsement by Dr. William Wilson, emeritus professor at Duke University:

> *Dave felt that the research he did would demonstrate the power of God in healing, and it has done just that. But mostly it has demonstrated the preventive medical aspects of a faith in the one true God.*

This statement is revealing in so many ways. It suggests quite clearly that Dr. Larson had an agenda he intended to pursue. It also ominously suggests that one specific religion is associated with health benefits.

The John Templeton Foundation merits such extensive consideration because it has provided the most support for promoting an integration of religion and health. But Templeton is not alone in this effort. Other foundations and organizations also have provided support. The Fetzer Foundation, for example, has funded a number of initiatives on spirituality and medicine. The conservative lobbying organization Focus on the Family has provided support for Dr. Walter Larimore, who has written on the need to bring religion into medical practice. The RAMA Foundation, the Bakken Family Foundation, the George Family Foundation, and the FACT Foundation all provided support for the controversial MANTRA II study of distant, intercessory prayer (see Chapter 9).

The work of these foundations inspires grudging admiration. They set out to promote the idea that religion is good for your health, and they certainly have achieved that aim. In the middle of the first decade of the twenty-first century, this idea is widely accepted in the U.S.

## THE UNCRITICAL MEDIA

Much has been written about the change in news coverage in an era of corporate media ownership and consolidation. In the middle of the twentieth century, the news departments in broadcast media were distinct from the rest of their company. News was seen as a public service, and news departments were not encouraged to think about ratings or concern themselves about making a profit; the rest of the company subsidized them.

That philosophy no longer prevails. Today all divisions of broadcast organizations are driven by profit motives. The obvious result of this change in emphasis is that producers, editors, and reporters are drawn to topics they believe will attract viewers. Coverage of the news has become less investigative and more sensational as the news divisions have become profit centers. More and more, stories become newsworthy simply because they are marketable. The same market considerations also apply to the print media.

There is little doubt that in the media, stories about religion sell. The *Newsweek* Education Program Web site (http://school.newsweek.com/online_activities/cover1.php) reports that in 2001, the magazine's issue with the cover story on Mormons sold 240,000 newsstand copies, in contrast to the issue with the Sopranos on the cover, which sold 158,000. In 2002, the issue with the cover story on the Bible and the Koran sold 203,000 copies, while the issue with the cover story on Silicon Valley sold only 90,000 copies. The site reports that cover stories about religious matters sell more issues of a magazine on the newsstand—in fact, they're generally among the top issues for the year. In 2005 alone, *Newsweek* had two cover stories on Christianity. Each of these two issues contained multiple, extensive reports of religious involvement in the U.S. Each was replete with statistics from recent surveys about the state of religiosity or spirituality in the U.S. today.

The discoveries of modern medicine also seem to be inherently interesting to the public and may be almost as popular as stories about religion. Between 2001 and 2004, *Time* magazine had thirty-seven cover stories on medical matters. Among the topics considered were stem cells, Alzheimer's disease, inflammation, women and heart disease, brain development, meditation, SARS, and diabetes. Clearly, there is a great appetite for news coverage of medicine and health.

In attempting to understand the appeal of the combination of these two topics for the media marketplace, I interviewed a number of journalists, in the print and broadcast media, who have covered developments in this area. In their view, the rise in interest in connecting religion and health derives from several sources. First, there has always been an interest among the general public about this topic, since we all confront illness and since so many of us are concerned about religious matters. This widespread interest is directly relevant to the new economics of the news business: it guarantees that stories about religion and health will be broadly appealing, an important consideration for reporters and editors. Health stories sell. Like political candidates, news organizations also conduct polls about the interests of their constituents. These polling data reliably identify religion and health as topics of interest.

Another factor that contributes to the media coverage of religion and health is the fact that millions of people have attempted to cope with serious illness by religious means, including praying, attending services, and reading scripture. This has created a fertile field for media coverage of the issue.

Market considerations therefore incline the media to cover religion and health separately as well as together whenever possible. Even so, the coverage leaves much to be desired. Far too often, it is insufficiently skeptical, preferring to accept statements by patients, doctors, and scientists without scrutiny. We saw in Chapter 3 how the rise of subjectivity compromised rationality in the late twentieth century. Nowhere is this clearer than in the media coverage of stories about religion and health.

Here's an example. On August 23, 1998, *USA Today* published a column by Dr. Gary Posner reporting that one month earlier, on July 25, *USA Today* contained an article whose first sentence read, "Maybe doctors should write 'go to church weekly' on their prescription pads." This statement struck Posner as suspicious, as though he had seen it before. Indeed he had, since "*USA Today* had simply republished verbatim an old Associated Press story from February 1996!" Both articles uncritically reiterated the claim by Dr. Dale Matthews that of 212 studies on religion and health that he had reviewed, 75 percent were positive. No effort to validate this claim was made either by the AP or the July 1998 *USA Today* journalist. According to Posner, a large proportion of the 212 articles cited by Matthews were written by parapsychologists way out of the scientific mainstream. As you'll see later, these claims about the number of studies demonstrating health benefits of religious practices are almost always grossly exaggerated.

This example illustrates not only the uncritical nature of *USA Today* and the AP but also the phenomenon of *metanarratives* that characterizes the press today. Metanarratives are stories that take on such significance that they themselves, instead of real news, spawn other news stories. That is, a reporter will file a story based not on information he or she has gathered but rather on some news already the basis of another news story. According to the Project on Excellence in Journalism, metanarratives are the modern equivalent of pack journalism.

*Pack journalism* refers to the tendency of reporters to collect in a group, look over the shoulders of other reporters as they file their stories, and then write the same story for their papers. Today, of course, reporters are far less likely to literally hang around in packs, but the effect may be the same nonetheless. In this era of electronic and Internet journalism, reporters may not look over each other's shoulders, because they can see on the Net what the others have written. And rather than expend the effort to investigate on their own, far too many take the easy way out and base their articles on "facts" that appear in other articles.

I experienced this phenomenon quite recently. A *Wall Street Journal* reporter who was writing an article on religious services and mortality contacted me. The article was a review of the scientific literature on this issue, not a story about a newly released study. Nevertheless, as a result of this media appearance, I received several other calls for interviews by journalists, simply because the *Journal* had covered this matter. Each of these interviews resulted in a story in another newspaper or magazine.

Another element of media coverage of religion and health is the reliance on anecdote to convey information and make a point. The cover story of the December 20, 2004, issue of *U.S. News & World Report* was devoted to the power of prayer. One of the articles recounted the following: "I was scheduled to have open-heart surgery for three blocked arteries in my heart. Friends and family prayed, and the next morning my doctor said my heart's arteries were as clear as a teenager's!"

This story was presented without comment, as though no examination was necessary. But precisely such an examination is absolutely essential to account for this highly improbable occurrence. Everything we know about coronary artery disease indicates that it does not disappear overnight. Even with powerful new medications like statins, coronary atherosclerosis recedes only over months. So it is extremely unlikely that this story can be correct. A responsible publication would at least have raised this issue.

Anecdotes are almost always interesting and are often compelling. That is undoubtedly why this story was included in the article. But as we'll see in detail in Chapter 6, anecdotes are not evidence. The case above tempts us to conclude that prayer and faith led to the reversal of this patient's heart disease. Even if we ignored the biology of coronary artery disease, the anecdote cannot be the basis of a medical conclusion, because we don't know how many people recovered in this way without prayer and increased faith, and how many people resorted to prayer but nevertheless didn't recover. If we had this kind of systematic evidence, we could validly draw a conclusion. The anecdote alone doesn't permit this.

## HISTORICAL "GREAT AWAKENINGS"

The role of religion in American society is constantly changing. For example, concerns about the appropriate relationship between church and state have always existed in the U.S., but at the turn of the twenty-first century, they are particularly pronounced. When John Kennedy ran for president in 1960, one of the most pressing issues in the campaign was whether his actions as president would be influenced by his Catholic faith. Kennedy had to assure the public that if he was elected, he would act on behalf of all Americans, not only Catholics. In a September 12, 1960, speech in Houston, candidate Kennedy said, "I do not speak for my church on public matters; and the church does not speak for me." He added,

> I believe in an America where the separation of church and state is absolute; where no Catholic prelate would tell the President—should he be Catholic—how to act, and no Protestant minister would tell his parishioners for whom to vote. . . . I believe in an America that is officially neither Catholic, Protestant nor Jewish; where no public official either requests or accepts instructions on public policy from the Pope, the National Council of Churches or any other ecclesiastical source; where no religious body

*seeks to impose its will directly or indirectly upon the general popu-
lace or the public acts of its officials.*

The contrast with politicians of today could not be greater. Rather than declare that their actions will be guided by the needs of all of those they represent, many of today's American politicians piously declare their faith to be one of their most significant attributes. The religious-political pendulum in America has swung to the opposite pole.

This kind of change in the role of religion in American society may be part of a larger pattern. According to economist Robert Fogel of the University of Chicago, religious enthusiasm in the U.S. is cyclical, with upsurges every hundred years or so. These "great awakenings," Fogel argues, consist of three phases. In the first, religious revival is characterized by increased intensity of religious belief and the establishment of new ethical principles that derive from these beliefs. The revival phase is succeeded by the implementation of political activity consistent with these ethical principles. These cycles end, Fogel argues, when these ethical and political activities are challenged and ultimately decline.

Fogel writes that a new great awakening, the fourth in U.S. history, began in the 1960s with "a revulsion with what believers see as the corruption of contemporary society. Believers in the new religious revival are against sexual debauchery, against indulgence in alcohol, tobacco, gambling, and drugs, against gluttony, and against all other forms of self-indulgence that titillate the senses and destroy the soul." Such a description perfectly characterizes the puritanical religious intensity that currently captures much of the U.S. It is also consistent with the conflation of medicine and morality, something discussed later in this book.

Fogel also describes the dissatisfaction with contemporary technological medicine we considered above. He writes that the fourth great awakening "is best understood as the most recent manifestation of the recurring effort to bring human institutions into some reasonable balance with the massive technological changes that periodically destabilize the prevailing culture."

We can debate the merits of Fogel's position, but there is little doubt that religious enthusiasm has waxed and waned throughout American history. As the speech from John Kennedy's 1960 campaign demonstrates, religion's role in American society then differed substantially from its role today. The rise in the belief that religion is linked to health, and should be linked to medicine, no doubt reflects the religious awakening we now confront.

Social movements do not arise in a vacuum. They are the product of cultural forces that shape their direction and character. The movement to bring religion into clinical medicine is no exception. As we have seen in this chapter, at least four factors may explain why, at the turn of the twenty-first century, this interest has flourished: the dissatisfaction with modern, technological medicine; the role of advocacy organizations; uncritical media; and the cyclical rise and fall of religious sentiments in the U.S. In the previous chapter, we considered the role played by the rise in irrationalism.

As Fogel's work suggests and as the history of other social movements demonstrates, the drive to link religion to medicine will eventually fade as it is eclipsed by something else. While that certainly is desirable, no one knows when this will happen and how much damage will be done to medicine in the meantime.

# PART TWO

Reading the Evidence

# 5

## ARE THERE REALLY SO MANY STUDIES
## ON RELIGION AND HEALTH?

**By the middle of the first decade of the twenty-first** century, there were thousands of studies in the scientific literature reporting connections between religious activity or involvement and health. Some suggest that religious activity protects against disease or enhances recovery. Some have suggested that attendance at religious services extends life: that people who go to church, synagogue, or other religious services more frequently live longer than those who attend less often or not at all. Along with the factors we considered in the previous chapter, these reports are responsible for the growing view that religious practices are good for your health.

Reviewers of this literature suggest that most of these studies show positive effects of religious involvement. Dr. Walter Larimore, sometimes associated with Focus on the Family, has written that "the vast majority of these cross-sectional and prospective cohort studies have shown that religious beliefs and practices are consistently associated with better mental and physical health outcomes." Other reviewers draw similar conclusions. Dr. Harold Koenig, the psychiatrist at Duke University, reports that more than 850 studies have examined the relationship between religious involvement and mental health, with over two-thirds reporting an advantage to the religiously involved. Regarding physical illness, he declares that of the more than 350 studies that examine connections to religious involvement, more than half show positive relationships. Mayo Clinic physician Paul Mueller and colleagues uncritically reproduce precisely this assertion: "A majority of the nearly 350 studies of physical health and 850 studies of mental health that have used religious and spiritual variables have found that religious involvement and spirituality are associated with better health outcomes." Dr. Dale Matthews, the internist at Georgetown University, and colleagues report that 80 percent of the published studies report a positive association between religious commitment and better health.

If these statements are any guide, there is a general consensus that (1) there are a great many studies on religion and health and (2) the majority of them show health benefits of religious involvement. However, the history of medicine and science is filled with hypotheses that ultimately were proven wrong through solid scientific research.

Consider the following examples:

- Early in the twentieth century, the accepted view about the causes of peptic ulcers held that diet, excessive gastric acidity, and local circulatory disturbances were responsible. By the 1940s, the view of ulcers had changed significantly: now psychosomatic factors were thought to be the cause, and virtually all experts agreed. Now we know that all of these views were wrong. The main cause of ulcers is an infectious agent, *Helicobacter pylori*. With this new understanding of the underlying causal mechanism, the approach to treatment changed as well. Now it is mainly pharmacological.
- For years, pediatricians routinely recommended that the healthy way for newborns to sleep was on their stomach. This advice was accepted universally. However, in 1992, the American

Academy of Pediatrics (AAP) recommended that all healthy infants younger than one year of age sleep on their back to reduce the risk of Sudden Infant Death Syndrome (SIDS). Since the AAP's recommendation, the rate of SIDS has dropped by over 40 percent.

- In the 1950s, a widely used surgical technique to treat severe coronary artery disease involved ligating, or tying off, the mammary arteries. The rationale for this procedure was that it would divert blood to the heart. Success rates for the procedure were substantial, with up to 95 percent of patients reporting that their heart disease symptoms had improved. But in 1959, a landmark paper in *The New England Journal of Medicine* reported that a double-blind trial of the procedure revealed it to be no more effective than sham surgery. That is, patients who merely had their chests opened and then closed, without ligating the mammary arteries, did just as well as those who had the full procedure. The publication of that paper led to abandoning a procedure that most had accepted as effective.

In each of these examples, medical procedures that were widely accepted as effective were shown by later research to be unsupported. Will the same be true of claims about the health benefits of religion?

## HOW MANY STUDIES ACTUALLY EXIST?

To determine how many studies exist, we need to make some distinctions. For example, it may be true that there are a great many studies on the topic of religion and health, but it may be equally true that many are not relevant to determining the health benefits derived by religiously involved people. That is, there may be scientific studies that look at *other* matters that are generally about religion and health but say nothing about health benefits of religious activity. In fact, there are a great many such studies.

## Studies of Denominational Differences

The scientific literature is full of reports from studies that examine denominational differences in health characteristics. That is, studies may show that the prevalence of heart disease is greater among Protestants than among Catholics, or that diabetes is more frequently found in Jews than in Christians or Muslims. Such studies comparing denominational differences are indeed about religion and health, but they are not about the benefits of religious involvement, since all the groups involved are religious. They just differ in their religious orientations.

Other studies vary this research strategy slightly. For instance, a number of studies from the 1960s and 1970s contrasted Seventh-Day Adventists or Mormons with other groups. Thus, for example, according to a report published in 1964, total cholesterol levels were lower across all age groups for a cohort of Seventh-Day Adventists compared to age-matched healthy New York City men and women. This is another study about religion and health that is unrelated to benefits of religious involvement. After all, we know nothing about the religiosity of the New York City residents.

The point of these studies was not to contrast groups differing in religiosity with each other. Rather, to take the last example, comparing Seventh-Day Adventists to residents of New York City was a way of examining the impact of differences in behavioral risk factors for disease. Seventh-Day Adventists are often studied precisely because their behavioral codes proscribe smoking and alcohol consumption. Making denominational comparisons like this is a convenient way of contrasting groups whose differing profiles of risk behaviors are of interest. Such comparisons have nothing to do with testing a health advantage of religious involvement. Anyone, religious or not, who followed these risk-reduction behaviors would have a health advantage.

# Studies Investigating the Impact of Health on Religious Involvement

We've all seen or heard about situations in which people adopt new religious habits as a result of becoming sick or injured. Sometimes the illness results in greater religiosity. But on other occasions, people lose their faith after they become sick. In either case, these are situations in which a person's religious involvement is the product of, rather than the cause of, a health condition.

Scientists are interested in this topic, too, and researchers have asked questions about the religious consequences of serious illness. For example, Dr. Jeff Levin found that mothers who were unhealthier, measured subjectively, prayed more for their babies. Healthier mothers prayed less for their babies. In another study, the impact of traumatic disability on changes in spiritual beliefs was examined. Among other findings, these authors reported differences in the spirituality expressed by patients with brain injuries and patients with spinal cord injuries. In both these studies, religious activities were the product of difficult life circumstances rather than factors that caused a health outcome.

Studies like these are not surprising, because many people turn to religious practices when threatened by medical problems. Such studies are common, and again, while they are about religion and health, they are irrelevant to concerns about the impact of such practices on health outcomes.

## Studies of Medical Decision Making

Many papers in the scientific literature address the influence of religious factors on medical decision making. For example, some religious denominations do not permit organ donation or blood transfusions. Attitudes toward end-of-life issues such as withholding of nutrition and hydration or advance directives and living wills also may vary considerably from denomination to denomination. Some Christian patients, for example, request aggressive medical interventions near the end of life, in contrast to others, who are willing to withhold hydration. Again, research studies on these topics are about religion and health but not about health advantages of religious involvement.

## Studies Only Remotely About Religion

Some papers in which measures of health and religion appear are only remotely about religious matters. For example, among the papers cited in comprehensive reviews of religion and health is one published in 1968 titled "Occupational Stress, Law School Hierarchy, and Coronary Artery Diseases in Cleveland Attorneys." Why is this study included in reviews of studies on religion and health? Because among the data reported was the fraction of the study sample that was Jewish. As the title suggests, this is not a paper about religion and health. Similarly, Dr. George Comstock reported data on church attendance in a paper entitled "Fatal Arteriosclerotic Heart Disease, Water Hardness at Home, and Socioeconomic Characteristics." Again, church attendance was only one of many variables measured. The same is true of many of these papers.

So it's clear that while there may be many research papers on religion and health, they may have nothing to do with the effect of religion on health. Biostatistician Emilia Bagiella and I attempted to determine more precisely how many studies were actually about a health advantage associated with religious involvement. We reviewed all studies in the medical literature appearing in the year 2000 that were identified as related to religion by Medline, an electronic database operated by the National Library of Medicine. It contains information on more than 12 million scientific articles in medicine, nursing, dentistry, veterinary medicine, and the health care system since the mid-1960s.

Each Medline entry contains basic information on the article, including an abstract or summary of the paper's background, methods, findings, and conclusions. Medline entries also contain keyword descriptions that allow the user to search for studies on specific topics. We searched the Medline database for all studies published in the year 2000 that were identified by a single keyword: "religion."

This very straightforward search yielded 266 papers. Dr. Bagiella and I then independently reviewed the abstracts of all 266 and classified them according to whether they were relevant to health benefits of religious activities. After reconciling differences between our two sets of reviews, we determined that only 42 of 266, i.e., 17 percent, were relevant to these claims. That's right—in the year 2000, there were 266 papers generally about religion and health, but only 17 percent of them were relevant to claims of health benefits of religious involvement. What were the remaining 83 percent of these studies about?

As expected, many of these studies were about denominational differences in health. Others were about the impact of health conditions on religious activities, that is, about whether people's religious behaviors and attitudes were caused by health problems. Others were about religious influences on physician behavior. Still others were about the impact of religious orientation on medical decision making. Some described health fairs conducted in churches.

Thus, the vast majority of the 266 papers that appeared in 2000 and were identified by Medline as relevant to religion and health were entirely irrelevant to claims that religion is good for your health. Of course, it's difficult to extrapolate from the literature in a single year to the entire literature. But it seems unlikely that the year 2000 was exceptional. There is no reason to believe that our findings would be any different if we had looked at 2001, 2002, or any other year.

So proponents of a connection between religion and health are technically correct when the write that there are a great many studies on the topic. But they are wrong when they report that the vast majority demonstrate positive relationships between religious involvement and better health. In fact, the vast majority of these studies have nothing whatsoever to do with the health benefits of religious involvement.

However, some studies do attempt to investigate possible health benefits of religious involvement. For these studies, we must ask the question: How good are they?

# 6

## HOW GOOD IS THE EVIDENCE?

To begin to determine the quality of studies relating health benefits to religious involvement, let's consider one of the earliest and largest, conducted by Dr. George Comstock from the Department of Epidemiology at Johns Hopkins University in Maryland. Hopkins is one of the world's most renowned medical institutions. As an index of its prestige, it receives more funding from the National Institutes of Health than any other university in the country.

The Department of Epidemiology at Hopkins is the oldest in the world, and it has been at the forefront of research into the causes of diseases from cancer to infectious diseases to HIV/AIDS. At the time of these studies and since then, Dr. Comstock has been a leading epidemiologist. Throughout his illustrious career, he has received a great many academic and professional awards.

Epidemiologists ask questions about the factors that determine health and disease of human populations. Generally, they attempt to answer these questions using large data sets that contain information about people and their families, work, interests, and environments, among other factors. This information is collected from a great many people, usually thousands at a time. Epidemiologists sift through this information to examine relationships between variables that are of interest to them. For example, the first evidence of the health risks of smoking came from epidemiological studies showing that people who smoked cigarettes had substantially higher rates of cancer and heart disease than nonsmokers.

In 1963, nearly one hundred thousand residents of Washington County, Maryland, were surveyed and completed interviews with representatives of Johns Hopkins, the National Cancer Institute, and the Washington County Department of Health. They were asked a series of questions about many aspects of their lives and their health. Some of the questions were about how frequently they attended religious services: Did they attend services at least once a week? One or two times a month? Only once a month? Less frequently still? Never?

In the 1970s, Comstock began to analyze this large data set. He was interested initially in whether there was a relationship between attendance and heart disease mortality. To answer this question, he and his colleagues then established who was still alive and who had died three to five years after completing the survey. He then compared these two groups, those who survived and those who had died, on the frequency of attendance at religious services and concluded that there was a direct relationship between attendance and survival. The more frequent the attendance reported in 1963, the more likely it was that the respondents were still alive at the time the follow-up was conducted.

Epidemiologists typically report the findings of their studies in *risk ratios* that express the likelihood that one group relative to another will develop a disease. We all accept the fact that smoking increases the risk of having a heart attack. Risk ratios help us to understand *how much* the risk is increased. For example, a recent study revealed that among thirty-five- to thirty-nine-year-old women, the risk ratio of a nonfatal heart attack was 5.3 for women who smoke. This means that in women, smokers in this age range are about five times more likely to have a nonfatal heart attack than nonsmokers. The risk ratio for men was about the same.

Comstock reported a risk ratio of about 2, meaning that the death rate among the infrequent attenders was about twice that of those who attended more frequently. But was the finding real? Was there really a relationship between attendance at services and mortality? And if so, did it mean that attending services could extend your life? Some people certainly believe that this is true. But in this case, they probably are wrong.

To find out why, we need to consider how science operates. As we saw in Chapter 3, science is an organized way of gathering information and establishing relationships among objects and events in the universe. A fundamental principle of science is its reliance on observation as a source of information. Scientific knowledge depends upon observable and testable facts.

Our review of the history of religion and medicine showed that until the sixteenth century, this approach to knowledge was uncommon. Knowledge—religious, scientific, philosophical, or political—derived primarily from the authority of the Church. The Italian astronomer Galileo achieved fame, but also notoriety, by challenging this view. He promoted observation and experimentation as the way to acquire information. His support for the Copernican view of the solar system—that the Earth revolved around the Sun and not vice versa—led to his official condemnation by the Church because this view was contrary to the biblical one. Nonetheless, Galileo persisted in promoting observation rather than authority as the primary source of knowledge, so the Church imprisoned him in 1633. Authority as the primary source of knowledge may have won that battle, but it lost the war. Galileo's views came to be recognized as a fundamental principle of science, one that we still hold today. Galileo was one of the first true scientists in the modern sense of the word. Observation of events is the cornerstone of contemporary science. But at the beginning of the twenty-first century, we again see religious authority challenging this view.

# ANECDOTE VS. EVIDENCE

But observation alone may not be a sufficient source of scientific knowledge. Scientific observations, as we saw earlier, must also be *systematic*. That is, they must be collected in a way which ensures that they are representative of the phenomenon in question. Anecdotes also may be based on observation, but they are not evidence. Anecdotal accounts of events, unless accompanied by systematic observations, may be highly misleading.

Consider this very current example: in these days of alternative medicine, claims are often made about the health benefit of vitamins or herbs. It may be true that a friend felt a cold coming on and took the herbal remedy echinacea, and the cold never arrived. Is this scientific evidence that echinacea prevents colds?

Absolutely not. As an anecdote, this is an acceptable account of this individual's experience. As a scientific observation, however, it has little value. Why?

There are two reasons: (1) We have no idea how many other people felt a cold coming on and did precisely the same thing (took echinacea) but still came down with a cold, and (2) we also have no idea how many people felt a cold coming on and did nothing at all but nevertheless did not come down with a cold. In medicine, there are a great many conditions that get better by themselves with no intervention whatsoever. This is spontaneous remission, a matter we covered in Chapter 3.

An anecdote is not evidence. It may be interesting, even compelling, but it is nothing more than one person's account of an event. The only way to determine definitively and scientifically that echinacea prevents colds is to *systematically* study people who feel a cold coming on, and randomly give half of them echinacea and the other half a harmless sugar pill or placebo, then follow them for a week to determine whether these two groups develop colds at a different rate. That is, we would conduct an experiment or a randomized trial. The key here is to *randomly* assign subjects to receive echinacea or a placebo so that we can be certain that the two groups don't differ in ways that might influence the likelihood of getting a cold. For example, if instead of randomly assigning subjects, we allowed people to select whether they wanted to receive echinacea or not, we could bias the results because those who chose echinacea might be more likely to approve of alternative medicine and expect it to work. So they would be less likely to report catching a cold.

If we conducted the study properly and discovered that the echinacea group developed fewer colds than the placebo group, we'd be justified in concluding that echinacea prevented colds. *Systematic* and unbiased data collection is the key. We need to rule out all competing explanations for our findings. If we can't do that, we can't conclude anything. Ironically, a recent report described precisely this study of echinacea and demonstrated quite conclusively that it did not work.

Anecdotal accounts of the effectiveness of religious activities appear all the time in the media. But such anecdotes have no more value than the anecdote about echinacea and colds. A noteworthy example comes to mind.

## THE CASE OF ELIZABETH SMART

We frequently read stories in the newspaper or see stories on the evening news that tell us about the role that prayer or religion has in making a bad situation better. Because they are truly compelling and heartwarming, the truth of these stories is rarely questioned. One of the most famous of these recent stories, the kidnapping of Elizabeth Smart, has a direct bearing on the way we think about the power of prayer. Although her story is not related to health per se, it nevertheless tells us something important about how those involved in the case saw the effect of prayer, and how the media presented it.

In 2002, teenager Elizabeth Smart disappeared from her home in Utah. After nearly a year, she was recovered in a nearby town, apparently the victim of abduction by a self-described prophet. Her father remarked that "the prayers of the world have brought Elizabeth home," and her uncle said, "I don't think any little girl was prayed for more in the history of the world."

Without a doubt, Elizabeth Smart's father and uncle were comforted by the prayers of others, and we shouldn't diminish the importance of this. But just as in the case of echinacea and colds, the conclusion that she was recovered alive and well because of the prayers of others is simply an anecdote. Just as in the case of echinacea, we have no idea how many other girls are abducted every year, are the recipients of the prayers of a great many people, but are never recovered; and we have no idea how may girls are abducted and are recovered despite little prayer on their behalf.

We do know, however, how many girls are abducted and never recovered. Extrapolating from 1999 data from the U.S. Department of Justice, during the year that Elizabeth Smart was held captive there were an estimated 58,200 child victims of nonfamily abduction. An estimated 46 percent of these kidnapping victims were sexually assaulted, and an additional 31 percent were physically assaulted. Some were killed and some were never recovered.

Do we really believe that there were no prayers for the kidnapped children who were killed or injured? And are we certain that all of the children who were returned home safely were the recipients of prayer?

Anecdotal accounts more specifically related to the health benefits of religion also appear with great regularity, not only in the news media but also in books by physicians. For instance, *The Faith Factor* by Dr. Dale Matthews is laced with heartwarming anecdotal accounts of medical cases in which patients succeed against all odds after religious interventions. Martha, we read, expected to die after a diagnosis of adenoid cystic carcinoma. Matthews informs us that physicians told her that her disease was terminal and that conventional cancer treatments would not help. After this diagnosis, Martha embarked on a series of alternative treatments, including a macrobiotic diet and a clinic for "exceptional cancer patients," neither of which worked. Then Martha, who had not been religious, started attending church and meeting with other church members for prayer and Bible study. She told the others about her condition, leading them to pray for her.

Nevertheless, the tumor did not disappear. Doctors recommended a new form of radiation treatment, but because of the severe side effects, Martha discontinued it after receiving only twelve of thirty-two sessions. Matthews reports that Martha informed the doctors that she was going to take her chances in the hands of the Lord. "Today, Martha is apparently in good health. The last MRI showed the tumor still in place, but Martha has no symptoms, and it has not grown."

By recounting Martha's case in this way, Matthews implies that it was her religious faith that was responsible for her unexpected survival. Unfortunately, as is always the case with these anecdotes, we lack the essential details to evaluate such a conclusion. For example, Matthews fails to tell us that adenoid cystic carcinoma is a very slow-growing cancer that rarely metastasizes to regional lymph nodes. We also don't know how long she has been followed since her radiation treatment—it could be only a few weeks or many years. Finally, we don't know with certainty that the abnormality on her most recent MRI actually was a tumor. As any radiation oncologist will tell you, an MRI scan without a biopsy reveals only the existence of a mass, not necessarily a tumor. The image on the MRI could be residual tissue that isn't cancerous, such as scar tissue produced by treatment or dead tumor cells. The only definitive way to know that the mass is a tumor is by biopsy. The possibility of noncancerous tissue is consistent with the report that the "tumor" had not grown, and with the fact that she had received approximately one-third of the new radiation therapy. The National Cancer Institute's Web site indicates that this treatment is effective for inoperable adenoid cystic carcinoma, and a paper published in 1991, seven years before Matthews published his book, demonstrated that the five-year survival rate with this treatment ranged from 65 percent to 93 percent. So perhaps Martha was still alive when

Matthews wrote his book because the cancer was slow growing or because the radiation treatment was effective. Because this account is only an anecdote, we can't say anything about this case for certain, least of all that her health was attributable to her religious devotion. If Dr. Matthews had really been more interested in evidence than advocacy, he'd have been more cautious in his presentation of this information.

To truly appreciate how misleading these anecdotes can be, consider the case of biologist Stephen Jay Gould, who was told in July 1982 that he had mesothelioma, a rare, incurable cancer with a median survival time of eight months after diagnosis. Such a statistic might have led others to despair, but Gould knew better. That is, he knew what the statistic meant: that half of those diagnosed with mesothelioma would be dead within eight months *but the other half would survive longer than eight months, possibly very much longer*. The survival curve looked something like this:

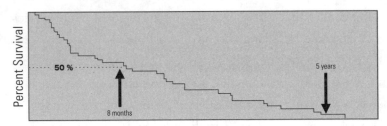

Hypothetical survival curve showing how half of patients with mesothelioma will live longer than the median survival time of eight months.

This figure shows that at eight months, 50 percent of the patients have died. But it also shows that 50 percent of the patients remain alive at eight months. And it shows that some patients will survive much longer than eight months. It's part of the natural variation of this disease.

In fact, Gould lived for twenty years after his diagnosis and died of another, unrelated cancer. The cases of Martha and Stephen Jay Gould illustrate nicely the problem with anecdotal accounts. They show that there is inherent variability in survival time after the diagnosis of a life-threatening disease. If we focus on only a single patient who fell on the rightmost part of the survival curve, we miss the fact that this was part of the normal variation in these cases, and we also have no idea if those patients on the left side of the curve—those patients who died sooner than expected—were also the beneficiaries of religious practices that supposedly enhanced their well-being.

Anecdotal observations play an important role in science. They often provide information that leads to the formulation of hypotheses that can be tested by standard scientific means. One of the most celebrated discoveries in the history of science was allegedly the product of an anecdotal experience: Newton's apple. According to the story, Newton was sitting beneath an apple tree when he saw an apple fall to the ground. This single experience led him to develop the law of gravity. Three hundred years later, this law still governs most of our physical world. Newton recognized that based on this single experience alone, no firm conclusions could be drawn. Only after formulating the law of gravity and testing it against observable facts was Newton able to say definitively that the trajectories of the planets and moons could be explained by gravity.

Alone, anecdotal accounts of events have little scientific value and can *never* be the basis of scientific conclusions. When you hear or read about such cases, remember how limited they are. Unless we *systematically* collect this information, we do not have evidence; all we have are anecdotes. Scientific conclusions require systematic observations.

But drawing conclusions becomes even more complicated because there are times when even systematic observation can mislead us. Our powers of observation are imperfect, and we may not see things as they truly are, not because we're careless but because things are complex. In Chapter 3, we saw how various factors like spontaneous remission can bias the scientific conclusions we draw. In research studies that employ an experimental design, these biases can be controlled. But in observational studies, as opposed to experiments, these approaches to controlling bias are not possible or are not effective. An aspect of American history provides us with a compelling and troubling example of this. It shows how observational studies can go very wrong, and it tells us something important about the Comstock study on church attendance and mortality.

## CONFOUNDS

In the 1920s, U.S. immigration policy was driven by the emerging science of intelligence testing. Although IQ tests were originally supposed to measure *acquired* characteristics, as they developed in the U.S., they were thought to measure *native* or *hereditary* intelligence. Therefore, it was thought that they could be used to characterize groups of people with different hereditary, and therefore presumably unalterable, intellectual attributes.

The 1920s were a time of rising xenophobia in the U.S. Foreigners were viewed with suspicion, especially those whose ethnicity differed from the ethnicities of the founders of the country. To address the rising influx of immigrants coming to the U.S., Congress passed a series of laws establishing a mechanism by which immigration could be regulated. These laws were heavily influenced by the new science of intelligence testing. IQ tests developed for the U.S. Army were used to establish an ethnic hierarchy of intelligence. At the top of the list were the Scandinavians, the English, and the Scottish. Europeans such as the French, Dutch, Belgians, and Germans were next. Below them were the Italians, Spanish, Hungarians, and Poles. And at the bottom of the list were Jews and blacks. This ethnic intelligence hierarchy led Congress to establish quotas that allowed much greater immigration by groups higher on the list than by those lower on it. Thus, immigrants of northern European extraction were favored over those from central or southern Europe, based on "scientific evidence" of differences in native intelligence.

How were these differences established? By the new science of

IQ testing. Here are some examples of the questions asked by these new tests:

Crisco is a: patent medicine, disinfectant, toothpaste, food product

The number of a Kaffir's legs is: 2, 4, 6, 8

Christy Mathewson is famous as a: writer, artist, baseball player, comedian

While it may seem obvious now, it was not obvious in the 1920s that these questions reflect familiarity with American culture rather than native intelligence. After all, you have to know about baseball, a uniquely American sport in the early twentieth century, to know that the answer to the last question is "baseball player." Thus, immigrant groups more familiar with American culture did better on the tests. A look at the chart below should give you an idea of why some immigrant groups might outperform others on these tests, revealing a fundamental flaw in the science of IQ testing as it related to immigration.

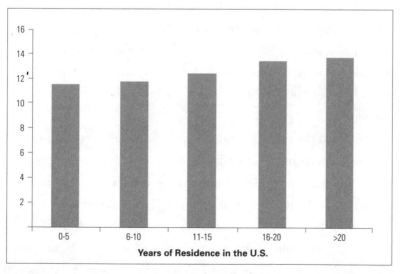

The impact of years residing in the United States on intelligence scores. Based on data presented by Gould, p. 221.

The chart makes clear that scores on intelligence tests were directly related to the amount of time that immigrant groups lived in the U.S. The longer an immigrant group resided in the U.S., the higher its members' IQ.

Now consider what historians of immigration have known for a long time: that immigration comes in waves, with groups of different origins arriving at different historical times. In the case of American immigration, the English and Scandinavians were among the earliest immigrants to the U.S. Later came the central Europeans, and after them the southern and eastern Europeans and the Jews.

It should be obvious by now that groups who have been in the U.S. longer will be more familiar with American culture and as a result will perform better on tests that really measure exposure to American culture rather than intelligence. Thus, the historical sequence of immigration to the U.S., not native intelligence, was responsible for the ethnic differences on IQ tests. It was not, as congressional representatives said at the time, that these groups differed in intelligence; rather, it was that they differed in exposure to American culture and therefore performed differently on IQ tests.

But the damage was done. As a result of laws passed by Congress in 1924, immigration by southern and eastern Europeans, which had begun to rise after 1890, fell sharply. The same Stephen Jay Gould whom we encountered above wrote that "we know what happened to many [of these would-be immigrants] who wished to leave but had nowhere to go."

So . . . what does this have to do with Comstock's finding of a relationship between church attendance and mortality? In the language of science, the years of residence in the U.S. is called a *confounder*. The purported relationship between ethnicity and IQ was *confounded* by time spent in the country. What was seen as ethnic differences in IQ was really attributable to the amount of time in the U.S. and the resulting familiarity with American culture. When we take into account the amount of time different ethnic groups spent in the U.S., the ethnic differences in IQ disappear entirely.

Is it possible that Comstock's study of attendance at religious services and mortality was similarly confounded? Comstock suggested that there was an inverse relationship between attendance and mortality, with those attending most frequently having the lowest mortality rates. Consider the relationship involved: those who survived until follow-up data were collected were more likely than those who died to have gone frequently to religious services. But people who attend services frequently *must be well enough to go frequently.* What if someone was unable to attend frequently because of poor health? People whose activities are limited by poor health may not be able to engage in a great many activities of daily living, including attending religious services.

But people who are in poor health are also, other things being equal, more likely than those in good health to die. Thus, the relationship Comstock found between attendance at religious services and mortality really was attributable, not to an effect of attendance on health, but rather to the fact that people who were too sick to attend services were also the ones who were most likely to die. Rather than religious attendance influencing health, it was health influencing attendance. In an article published several years later, Comstock acknowledged that this may have been the case. As we'll see later, more recent studies of attendance at religious services and mortality attempt to correct for this effect of poor health.

Confounding is a serious problem in this sort of research. It arises because almost all studies examining relationships between religion and health are *observational* in nature. They operate by observing subjects who already vary in the measure of interest, e.g., frequency of attendance at religious services, and then seek to examine differences between these groups on other measures of interest, in this case, health. In these kinds of studies—the only kinds that are possible in studies of religion and health—subjects *self-select* their religious activities. In a true experiment, such as a study of the effect of a new drug, an *experimenter* does the selecting, by assigning subjects on a random basis to either receive the new drug or not.

There have been some celebrated recent cases that illustrate the conflict between observational studies where self-selection is a concern and clinical trials. For example, several large epidemiology studies had provided evidence that women who selected estrogen replacement therapy were more protected against heart disease than women who did not. That is, women who took hormone replacement therapy (HRT), according to these observational studies, were less likely to develop heart disease than those who didn't. To confirm this relationship, several controlled trials were conducted. Everyone expected that the results of the trials would match the results of the observational studies. But when the trials were conducted, with random assignment of HRT or a placebo to groups of postmenopausal women, the findings were considerably different. Rather than providing protection for the women, hormone replacement actually *increased* their risk of breast cancer, stroke, and pulmonary embolisms.

Another celebrated conflict between observational studies and clinical trials involves the antioxidant vitamin beta-carotene. Observational studies showed that people who consumed diets with large amounts of this vitamin were less likely to develop lung cancer. An influential review of these observational studies suggested strong support for the hypothesis that dietary beta-carotene reduced the risk of lung cancer. Regrettably, the results of a large clinical trial based on these observational studies revealed that contrary to expectation, subjects taking beta-carotene had an 18 percent *increase* in lung cancer.

These two cases illustrate how different the results of observational studies and controlled trials can be, and they should provide a cautionary tale to those who want to make recommendations about medical practice from observational studies alone. The results of the trials suggested that the inferences drawn from the observational studies were wrong.

We can conduct both observational studies and randomized trials to test the effects of HRT and beta-carotene, but we can't do this with religion. We can't confirm observational studies with randomized trials. We can't *make* some people attend services frequently and make others attend less frequently and then examine their health ten years later, as we would do in a controlled trial. People self-select; they choose their level of attendance on the basis of their personal needs and interests. To study a relationship between attendance and health, all we can do is find people who already vary in their attendance patterns and compare them on health measures. The problem with this strategy is that by definition, people who choose different levels of attendance differ in their motivations for attendance. And they may differ in a great many other ways, some of which might influence their health. We can't tell whether it is the attendance or some of these other factors that influence health. As we saw in the case of the Comstock study, frequent attenders also differed from infrequent ones in their physical health, and it was their health, not their attendance at services, that was responsible for their mortality.

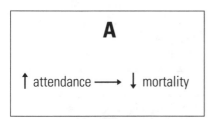

Figure A: The hypothetical relationship between attendance at religious services and mortality, suggesting that religiosity *causes* reduced mortality.

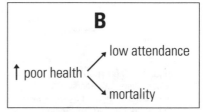

Figure B: The *more likely* relationship between attendance at religious services and mortality, indicating that poor health is linked to both lower rates of attendance and increased mortality.

Thus, the relationship depicted in Figure A is wrong. In the case of the Comstock study, the one in Figure B is correct.

We'll come back to the studies of attendance at religious services and mortality in a bit.

# MARKERS AND MECHANISMS

The lesson here is that in examining the observational studies of religion and health, it is essential to distinguish between factors that might actually cause health effects and those that are associated with these factors but don't actually influence health. We call these latter factors *markers*. The former factors, which actually are in the causal pathway to health, are called *mechanisms*. In the case of the Comstock study, attendance at services was merely a marker of poor health.

This distinction between markers and mechanisms is critical if our aim is to intervene to improve health or simply to predict health. For instance, it is very likely that the risk of Tay-Sachs disease is substantially greater among subscribers of *The New Yorker* than subscribers of *Christianity Today*. Is subscribing to *The New Yorker* a marker or a mechanism of Tay-Sachs disease? Do we believe that subscribing to *The New Yorker* causes Tay-Sachs, as depicted in Figure C?

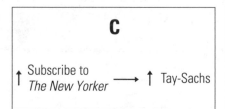

Figure C: The hypothetical relationship between subscribing to *The New Yorker* magazine and risk of contracting Tay-Sachs disease, suggesting that having a subscription *causes* the disease.

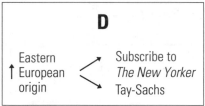

Figure D: The *real* relationship between subscriptions to *The New Yorker* and Tay-Sachs disease, showing that both are the product of ethnic origin

Of course not. These subscription patterns are simply markers of another factor, in this case a genetic one, that is responsible for the disease, as depicted in Figure D. Thus, it would be absurd to propose that we could eliminate Tay-Sachs by cutting off people's subscriptions to *The New Yorker*. We could use the marker to identify people at risk, but that would not tell us why they were at risk or how to reduce the risk.

A similar example involves the increased risk of heart disease associated with a crease that appears in the earlobe. Researchers have known about this peculiar fact for years. In a recent study, 85 percent of patients with heart disease also had a crease in their earlobe. But no one knows why this is so.

The example of the earlobe crease nicely illustrates the distinction between a marker and a mechanism. No one believes that the crease *causes* heart disease. It's not a mechanism, and it would be ridiculous to propose that we could treat heart disease by cutting off the earlobes of people who have creases in them. The crease is a *marker* of a disease process but is not causally involved in the development of heart disease. In many studies of religion and health, religious activities are more likely to be markers than mechanisms of good health.

## THE SHARPSHOOTER'S FALLACY

There is another kind of problem that characterizes the scientific literature suggesting relationships between religious activity and health. Physicist Robert Park of the University of Maryland refers to it as the "sharpshooter's fallacy." In this fallacy, the sharpshooter empties the six-gun into the side of the barn and *then* draws the bull's-eye around the bullet holes. Of course, in target shooting, you draw the bull's-eye first, then shoot. The same is true of science.

Robert Park is a trenchant critic of junk science. In the great tradition of physicists who go beyond their own narrow field of study to examine broader scientific, political, and social issues, Park has vigorously attacked what he calls "voodoo science." In his book by the same name, he provides instructive examinations of some of the great scientific frauds of recent times: cold fusion, perpetual energy machines, and quantum healing.

Examples of Park's sharpshooter's fallacy appear regularly in the literature on religion and health. A wonderful example, one that also illustrates some of the frustrations of conducting research in medicine, is provided by the research of the late psychiatrist Elisabeth Targ.

In the mid-1990s, Targ and her colleagues at the California Pacific Medical Center were investigating whether prayer and other forms of "distant healing" could be used to treat AIDS. Forty patients were recruited and randomly assigned to be in the treatment group and receive prayer and distant healing intentions from "experienced healers" around the country, or to be in the control group, which would receive only standard care. The healers included rabbis, Native American medicine men, and psychics.

The prayer treatment was spectacularly effective, according to the report of the study published in the *Western Journal of Medicine*. The control group, which didn't receive the prayers of the healers, contracted many more AIDS-related illnesses than the prayer group. They also stayed in the hospital much more than the prayer group. As a result of the study, Targ became famous instantly and appeared in many broadcast news shows, newspapers, and magazines.

But according to journalist Po Bronson, the story is not so simple. When Targ and her colleagues began the study, their aim was to see if the prayer treatment could have an impact on mortality. However, during the course of the study, the researchers were blindsided by the development of the then new antiretroviral therapies that revolutionized the treatment of AIDS. As a result, only one of the forty patients in their trial died, making it impossible to determine whether prayer had an impact on mortality. The researchers then sought to determine if the prayer treatment influenced some of their secondary outcomes such as physical symptoms, quality of life, mood, and counts of immune cells. It did not. Only after they analyzed length of stay in the hospital and physician visits did they find that the treatment and control groups differed in the predicted direction: the prayer group had shorter stays in the hospital and fewer visits to doctors.

This practice of contrasting two groups on one variable after another until a statistically significant difference emerges illustrates the sharpshooter's fallacy. Targ and her colleagues were drawing the bull's-eye after they had emptied the gun, violating a central principle of scientific investigation.

But this situation was even worse. As Bronson recounts it, after the researchers discovered the group differences on length of stay and physician visits, they were informed by another physician that these variables were not very interesting, because whether or not patients had health insurance heavily influenced these outcomes. Not surprisingly, patients with insurance were more likely to stay in the hospital longer and have more doctor visits. Health insurance, as we saw above, was a confounder.

Following the recommendation of this physician, Targ and colleagues then sought to determine whether their two groups of patients differed on twenty-three AIDS-related illnesses that had been identified in a very recently published paper. Unfortunately, these illnesses had not been measured in the original study, so the researchers, after already knowing which patients were in the treatment and control groups, went back to the charts to collect information on them. It was this information that they presented in their *Western Journal of Medicine* paper. There was no mention of the failure of distant healing to influence many of the original measures. Nor did the researchers mention that they had assessed AIDS-related illnesses after knowing which patients were in each group.

Thus, Targ and colleagues kept measuring outcome variables until they found some that distinguished between the prayer and the control groups. When they did, they stopped searching and published the paper. It's hard to find a better example of the sharpshooter's fallacy. You can't miss hitting the target if you draw the bull's-eye after unloading the gun.

Such poor research is not limited to Targ's study. Her paper is only one of many claiming to show a relationship between religious activity and health that make this fundamental mistake. In another, one by Harold Koenig and colleagues, researchers measured over 126 medical indicators before reporting that participants who attended church more frequently had lower blood pressures than those who attended less frequently. This paper is discussed in more detail later, but for now, consider that for almost all the other 126 variables they measured, there were no differences between frequent and infrequent attenders. This is not like using a six-gun on the side of a barn. It's like using an AK-47, and it's scientifically unacceptable. In science, you establish in advance what effects you believe your treatments will have, and then you determine whether you were correct, just as in target shooting, you establish the position of the bull's-eye, *then* fire the gun.

Sometimes the violation isn't so obvious. Consider an article by Hughes Helm and colleagues from Duke University about *private* religious behavior, such as Bible study, prayer, and meditation, in contrast to the more *public* behavior of attending religious services. This article reported that private religious behavior was not associated with a reduced risk of death among 3,851 elderly research subjects. That should have been the end of the story. But the researchers then went on to divide the sample on the basis of functional impairment, the same variable that Comstock and colleagues had found to be critical in their study. Helm and colleagues then reported that while there was still no relationship among subjects with impairments, there was a relationship among those who had no impairments. That is, those subjects who at entry into the study engaged in private religious behavior and were functionally intact lived longer than those who did not engage in private religious behavior and were functionally intact. For those who already had impairments, there was no such benefit.

On the surface, this study seems acceptable, but we are left with a nagging question: What led the researchers to divide the sample by functional impairment? Was it because in studies like Comstock's, it had been shown to be important? Although that was true, functional impairment was important in the Comstock study because it limited the capacity to get out of the house and attend religious services. *But it has nothing to do with private religious behavior like reading the Bible.* Whether functionally impaired or not, people can read the Bible.

Why did they choose this variable and no others? Why not divide according to gender? Or race? Or age? Or income? Or any number of other variables? Although we can't know for sure, in all likelihood, this is precisely what the researchers did, and they reported only the factor that produced the significant finding: functional impairment. Although more subtle than the Koenig paper that reported over 126 different statistical tests, this paper also is likely to have committed the sharpshooter's fallacy.

In science, this kind of *exploration of data* is not only appropriate but essential for hypothesis generation. But that is different from presenting this research as confirming an effect. The proper course of action would have been to report that an exploratory analysis of these data suggested that functional impairment might be an important variable to examine in relation to a possible association between private religious behavior and mortality and then to go on to test this *specific hypothesis* in a new study with a new sample of subjects.

## MULTIPLE COMPARISONS

Consider this example: you're flipping a coin and it seems to come up heads more frequently than seems reasonable. You might say to yourself, "Hey! This coin is fixed." But how would you know for certain? If it wasn't fixed, the probability that it would come up heads is 50 percent, i.e., 1 out of 2. On the basis of this probability, we'd expect that if we flipped the coin twice, it would, on average, come up heads once and tails once. If we flipped it 4 times, the result would be 2 heads and 2 tails.

But of course there is a chance, or a probability, that if it was flipped twice, it could come up heads on each flip. The probability of this is easily calculated. On any given coin toss, the probability of heads is $\frac{1}{2}$ or 50 percent. The probability of heads is $\frac{1}{2}$ on each toss, so if we flip it twice, the probability of two heads is $\frac{1}{2} \times \frac{1}{2}$, or $\frac{1}{4}$. Correspondingly, the probability of 4 heads on 4 flips is $\frac{1}{2} \times \frac{1}{2} \times \frac{1}{2} \times \frac{1}{2}$, or $\frac{1}{16}$, which is 6.25 percent. So it's unlikely that a coin would come up heads 4 times in 4 tosses, but there is a real, although small, chance that this could happen, even if the coin isn't fixed.

The question for us is what standard we will employ to determine whether the coin is fixed. After all, extrapolating from the above example, we can see that no matter how many times we flip the coin, there is a chance that it will come up heads on every flip even if it isn't fixed. The chance is real but very small, and it becomes smaller as the number of flips increases.

So here's the problem: How can we know whether 4 heads in 4 flips is the result of chance or a fixed coin? The answer is that we can *never* entirely rule out chance. Even 25 heads in 25 flips is possible, but it is very, very, very unlikely. The best that we can do is to agree upon a standard to determine *just how* unlikely an event must be for us to decide that it could not be the product of chance and must, therefore, be real.

In science, this standard has been established: we regard a finding as real if we determine that it would occur by chance less than 5 percent of the time. In our example above, we saw that the probability of getting 4 heads in 4 coin tosses was 6.25 percent. This exceeds the 5 percent standard that science has established, so we accept the fact that this result is the product of chance and reject the hypothesis that the coin was fixed. But if we flipped it 5 times, and on each occasion it came up heads, the probability would be $\frac{1}{2} \times \frac{1}{2} \times \frac{1}{2} \times \frac{1}{2} \times \frac{1}{2} = \frac{1}{32}$, which equals 3.13 percent. This is below the 5 percent standard, leading us to reject chance as an explanation—it's just *too improbable*—and accept that the coin is fixed.

What happens if instead of testing a single coin, we test two, each with a set of 5 flips? What are the odds that *one* of the two coins will come up heads 5 times by chance alone?

These odds are still very small, but they now are increased because we are flipping two coins: instead of the chance being 3.13 percent, it now is 6.15 percent.* In fact, each time we add another set of 5 coin flips, we increase the likelihood of getting 5 heads on one of the sets.

Now you can see why the sharpshooter's fallacy is not only unfair but profoundly misleading. We've tested so many coins that one of them is likely to produce 5 heads in 5 tosses by chance alone, *even if it's not fixed.* If we flip enough of them, we're certain that one set of 5 flips will yield 5 heads.

When a researcher tests the likelihood that a single finding is real, we accept it as real if we determine that it occurs by chance less than 5 percent of the time. We saw that when we add first one coin, then another, and another, the odds of an unlikely event—getting 5 heads in 5 flips—increase with each coin we add. In an identical fashion, when we test one variable, then another, then a third, and so on, the likelihood of one of them achieving the 5 percent standard increases with each new test we conduct. If we conduct enough tests, one certainly will reach that standard.

What we have done by conducting multiple tests is to lower our standards for determining whether a finding is real or the product of chance. That is, we increase our likelihood of *mistakenly calling a chance finding a real one.*

In the case of the coins, this means declaring the coin to be fixed when it's not. In the case of examining the relationship between a religious practice and health, e.g., church attendance and blood pressure, it may mean accepting that this relationship is real when it's not.

To take a hypothetical example, if we test the relationship between

---

*If you're interested, here's how to compute this probability: as we indicated above, the probability of 5 heads in 5 flips is 3.13 percent (or 0.0313). Correspondingly, the probability of getting any other combination of heads and tails in this set of 5 flips is 96.87 percent ($1 - 0.0313$). We're conducting two sets of 5 flips each, so there's the probability, although extremely small, of getting 5 heads on each of the two sets of 5 flips. This probability is $0.0313 \times 0.0313$. So the probability of getting one set of 5 heads in 5 flips when flipping the coin for two sets of 5 flips is $[(2 \times 0.0313 \times 0.9687) + (0.0313)^2] = 0.0615$ or 6.15 percent.

attendance and systolic blood pressure, diastolic blood pressure, mean arterial pressure (a kind of average of systolic and diastolic pressure), and pulse pressure (the difference between systolic and diastolic pressure), we increase the likelihood that one of these associations will reach the 5 percent threshold by chance alone. What if we not only test the relationship between these blood pressure variables and church attendance but also combine this with other indices of religiosity, e.g., reading the Bible, daily prayer, watching religious television, or listening to religious radio programming? Each of these additional variables means additional statistical tests, and each added test increases the chance that we'll make a mistake, confusing a chance finding for a real one.

One solution to this problem of conducting repeated statistical tests is to adjust our standard of certainty for distinguishing between a chance and a real finding. If, as in biomedical science, you accept the 5 percent criterion as the standard, then if you make only a single comparison, no adjustment is necessary. But if you make two comparisons, you have doubled the chance of achieving a difference between groups that reaches the 5 percent criterion. That is, you now accept a finding as real if it is likely to occur 10 percent of the time. And if you make four comparisons, you double the chance again, and accept a finding as real if it is likely to occur 20 percent of the time. Sooner or later, you make enough comparisons to guarantee that one will reach that 5 percent criterion. To correct for this problem, you can simply divide the 5 percent criterion by the number of comparisons you plan to make. If you plan to make two comparisons, you set your standard for statistical significance at 2.5 percent (5 percent ÷ 2). Three comparisons? 5 percent ÷ 3, or 1.67 percent, and so on.

This problem occurs over and over in the literature on religion and health, and far too often, researchers fail to make this simple adjustment in their criterion for statistical significance. My favorite example is the paper by Koenig and colleagues in which they examined whether religious involvement was associated with lower blood pressure. That's a reasonably straightforward question to ask, but Koenig et al. kept testing and testing until they found some significant differences between groups. They examined the relationship between attendance at religious services and whether, in 1986, participants reported that they had ever been told that they had high blood pressure. They examined this same relationship for data collected in 1989–90. And again in 1992–93. In 1986, they asked about the relationship between private prayer, meditation, or Bible study and whether participants had been told they had high blood pressure. Then again in 1989–90. And again in 1992–93. Then they asked about watching religious TV or listening to religious radio programming and being told of high blood pressure in 1986, 1989–90, and 1992–93. Then they asked precisely the same questions, but this time, instead of asking about whether participants had been told that they had high blood pressure, the researchers actually measured blood pressure. For data collected in 1986, 1989–90, and 1992–93. For both systolic and diastolic blood pressure. They broke the sample apart and looked at blacks and whites separately, and asked precisely the same questions. They did the same thing for older and younger participants.

I stopped counting the number of comparisons they made at 126. Koenig and colleagues claimed that their study showed that religiously active participants tended to have lower blood pressures. Of all the comparisons they made, only a very small number were claimed to be significant. If we looked at only these, we'd take this claim seriously, but we know that at least 126 separate tests were made. When we consider all of them, it's not surprising that some might, by chance, appear to show real differences between the groups. Looking at all of them, we know that the differences that appeared were most likely the products of chance.

These researchers could have considered their findings to be purely exploratory and then constructed very specific hypotheses to be tested in another research study. If they had done this and still found these relationships, they would be entitled to conclude that attendance at religious services was associated with lower blood pressure. But they didn't do this, so they can't draw this conclusion.

So what have we learned thus far?

- Anecdotes are not evidence—no matter how compelling, how heartfelt, how dramatic they are, anecdotes are unsystematic observations that may be highly misleading and do not represent other similar events. Scientific conclusions require systematic data collection.
- Studies that rely on observing already existing differences in participants may be misleading because they are at risk for confounding. Comstock's finding that church attendance was associated with reduced mortality was confounded by the failure to consider functional status.
- Factors associated with health outcomes may merely be markers of the risk and not causally linked to a disease. The earlobe crease is the perfect example. Attendance at religious services also may be a marker of some *other* factor that influences health.
- Scientific conclusions cannot be the products of the sharpshooter's fallacy. If you conduct enough comparisons in a study, you will almost certainly come up with a finding that achieves "significance," but that conclusion will be invalid.

Keep these facts in mind when you next hear about links between religious involvement and health.

We'll use these conclusions to evaluate studies that claim to show how religious involvement benefits health as we finally answer our second question: How good *are* the studies that are concerned with the health benefits of religion? But before we do that, let's examine some tricks of the scientific trade.

# 7

## IS THERE REALLY A HEALTH ADVANTAGE TO THE RELIGIOUSLY ACTIVE?

**Once a scientific study has been completed, the find**ings generally are reported. The way in which they are reported can give us a clue about how much confidence we should place in those findings. It's one of those areas in which the old dictum "Consider the source!" holds true.

## PUBLICATION, PRESENTATION, OR PRESS CONFERENCE?

One important question to ask yourself when you read or hear of a claim about a medical matter in general or about religion and health specifically is, what is the source of this claim? Although you may read about it in a newspaper or magazine or hear about it on the news, the original source may be an article published in a scientific journal, a presentation at a scientific meeting, a press conference, or a combination of all three.

The source, it turns out, is significant. Scientific information is not only acquired in a specific manner, as we saw above when discussing how to determine definitively whether echinacea prevents colds, but it is also disseminated in a specific way. Scientists publish their findings in peer-reviewed journals. That is, they write a manuscript reporting their findings and submit it to a journal that in turn asks other scientists with expertise in the area to evaluate it. These *peer reviewers* may find the research compelling and important or uninteresting and poorly conducted. They may recommend the manuscript for publication without change, may express support for the manuscript but recommend some modifications, may criticize it harshly but allow the authors to make the changes they recommend and resubmit it, or they may reject it altogether because they don't think the study was well conducted. This process of peer review is central to the scientific enterprise, and only those findings that make it through this process can qualify as scientific information. Only after findings are published in reputable, peer-reviewed journals do we consider them real scientific facts.

Of course, scientists also regularly attend professional meetings at which they present findings that have not yet been published, and the media often report on them. Even though presentations at scientific meetings are submitted to peer review, the standards for presentation are far less rigorous than those for publication. Only limited information on the research study is submitted to scientific meetings for possible presentation. That is, researchers usually submit only an *abstract* to the meeting organizers. An abstract is a brief summary of the research question, the methods, the findings, and the conclusions. Because it is so brief, it is impossible for the reviewers to understand the complete details of the study. For example, because the abstract is brief—generally less than 250 words—it may not contain information about confounding or the sharpshooter's fallacy. So it is possible for findings of relatively poor quality to be presented at scientific meetings. The level of review of findings submitted to meetings is not the same as when they are submitted for publication.

Finally, some scientists make their findings public at press conferences. In some cases, these press conferences are associated with the publication of a paper in a scientific journal, so the evidence reported at the press conference can be assumed to have been subjected to the rigorous evaluation of peer reviewers. But every once in a while, scientists go directly to the media with their findings, without bothering with the tedious but essential peer-review process. According to Robert Park of *Voodoo Science,* if scientists make their claims directly to the media, it's a sure signal that they do not have a finding that can survive peer review. That is, it's certain that the findings are highly questionable.

Here is an excellent example of this practice. On June 15, 2005, *The New York Times* reported that the Heritage Foundation had just released the findings of two new studies they had supported demonstrating that young people who took virginity pledges had lower rates of acquiring sexually transmitted diseases and engaged in fewer risky sexual behaviors. These findings were newsworthy because they contradicted previous findings that indicated that such pledges had no effect. However, it turned out that this report was not based on findings from a published paper. Rather, it was based on analyses that had not yet even been submitted for publication. Nevertheless, they merited a major news article in a major U.S. newspaper and, no doubt, coverage in the broadcast media, too.

The problem with the presentation of these findings is that they haven't been exposed to the peer-review process. Therefore, we have no details about the methods used by the researchers or whether they committed any of the errors we considered earlier. Without this information, we don't know whether we should have any confidence in these findings. Scientific findings reported in press conferences alone should be viewed with extreme skepticism.

## SPINNING THE MANTRA

Another, more complicated example of reporting through the media comes from the MANTRA study. MANTRA is an acronym for Monitoring and Actualization of Noetic Trainings. The full name is as opaque as the acronym, chiefly because of the odd word *noetic*. MANTRA principal investigator Dr. Mitchell Krucoff and colleagues define *noetic* as "a treatment discipline whose influence purports to enable, release, channel, or connect an intellectual, intuitive, or spiritual healing influence without the use of a drug, device, or surgical procedure." In other words, Krucoff and his colleagues were engaged in a study of some healing processes wherein no one—not a doctor, technician, or nurse—actually prescribes medicine, or uses a medical device.

In the late 1990s, Krucoff and colleagues initiated the MANTRA pilot study. The research subjects in this first effort were 150 patients who had chest pain at rest and were scheduled to receive either a diagnostic cardiac catheterization or an angioplasty. In both of these procedures, a catheter is snaked through a blood vessel and into the heart. In the diagnostic procedure, a dye is injected into the blood vessels of the heart to identify regions where these vessels are occluded. In angioplasty, an occluded blood vessel is unblocked, typically by inflating a small balloon at the tip of the catheter to compress the blockage against the artery wall. In the MANTRA pilot study, the following noetic techniques were used in addition to angioplasty:

1. Imagery
2. Touch therapy
3. Stress relaxation
4. Distant intercessory prayer
5. Standard care

In the group using imagery techniques, participants were taught to focus on a preferred place, one which was peaceful or relaxing, during a fifteen-minute session prior to the angioplasty. Some participants concentrated on warm sunny beaches, others on snowy mountains, still others on green meadows. After the angioplasty procedure was completed, the patients were encouraged to continue imagining this place.

Touch-therapy sessions for those in the second group lasted thirty minutes and were administered immediately prior to the angioplasty. The patients were taught to breathe slowly, focusing on abdominal breathing. Then the noetic therapist "gently touched the patient with both hands in the prespecified sequence of positions." There were twenty-two such positions throughout the body, each of which received approximately forty-five seconds of touch from the therapist.

Details about the stress-relaxation sessions are sketchy, but we know that they lasted thirty minutes, that patients received "instructions in self-relaxation skills," and that they were taught the same abdominal-breathing technique that the touch-therapy patients received. This breathing exercise was combined with a personally selected word or phrase that conveyed a sense of relaxation to the patient. Patients were asked to practice these relaxation exercises before the angioplasty.

In the distant-prayer condition, patients' names, illnesses, and procedures were provided to twelve prayer groups participating in the study. Among those included were a Baptist congregation in North Carolina; the Unity School of Christianity in Missouri; monastic centers in North Carolina, France, and Nepal; and a Virtual Jerusalem Web site in Israel. These groups prayed in whatever way they were accustomed to, from five to thirty days after each subject was enrolled. At no time were they in contact with the patients in any way.

In the standard-care condition, the patients received no special treatment. They were simply treated as usual. Krucoff and colleagues then compared these five groups on a number of outcome variables.

The results of the MANTRA pilot study were published in the *American Heart Journal* in 2001. Krucoff et al. reported that not one of the many medical outcome variables they collected was statistically significant. It didn't matter if the participant thought about the beaches of Nantucket, hummed "Claire de Lune" in his head, repeated the word *aquamarine* over and over, or was prayed for by a congregation in Nepal. No matter what the outcome variable, the treatment groups did not differ from each other in a significant way.

Even though the results were not significant, the undeterred MANTRA researchers went on to report a variety of nonsignificant differences between the groups. They reported that there was a 25 to 30 percent reduction in all outcomes in the four noetic treatment groups compared to standard care. They added further that among the noetic groups, the lowest level of adverse outcomes during hospitalization occurred in the prayer group. They also reported that all of the deaths in the study occurred in the noetic groups. But as indicated above, none of these differences was significant (a fact that was often obscured in these reports). That is, they could easily have been the result of chance alone. In a pilot study, it's perfectly appropriate to consider findings that don't achieve statistical significance as the basis for planning a larger, more definitive study. In fact, that's precisely the purpose of a pilot study. But it's not appropriate to discuss these nonsignificant findings as though they were meaningful. Krucoff appears to have done both, as we'll see below.

Buoyed by these findings, Krucoff began a much larger study, MANTRA II, in which 748 patients undergoing elective coronary interventions at nine centers around the U.S. were randomly assigned to receive one of four treatments:

1. Standard care
2. Distant intercessory prayer
3. A combination of music, imagery, and touch therapy
4. Both the combined therapy and prayer

MANTRA II sought to determine the survival rates of individuals in the different groups six months after they entered the study. MANTRA II was to be a *definitive* study. That is, it was designed to overcome the limitations of the MANTRA pilot study: too few subjects, enrollment of subjects at only a single site, a focus on men only, and the failure to assess the effect of combining noetic therapies. Because MANTRA II was big enough to draw firm conclusions, enroll women as well as men at many different sites in the U.S., and administer noetic therapies alone and in combination with each other, the investigators believed that it would provide definitive results about the effectiveness of these therapies.

The results of the MANTRA II study were not published until July 2005. We'll discuss the details in Chapter 9, but now it's important to focus on comments made about MANTRA II prior to publication, when the findings were unavailable for review. At an October 2003 conference on the use of complementary and alternative medicine in cardiology, sponsored by the American College of Cardiology, Krucoff revealed that the results of MANTRA II were similar to those from the MANTRA pilot study: groups that received the alternative treatments, either alone or in combination with each other, did not do any better than the groups that received standard medical care. As in the MANTRA pilot study, the prayer group did no better than the combined-treatment group or the standard-care group. The difference between the MANTRA pilot study and MANTRA II was that the latter was a much bigger study involving many more participants. It was big enough that if the noetic treatments really had an effect, they should have been apparent. But they weren't.

The BBC TV program *Everyman* reported these findings on October 23, 2003. In the press release for the program, Dr. Krucoff was quoted as saying, "The most basic data tables are negative; there is no difference." The story was picked up by many newspapers. This should have been the end of the story—no support for the hypothesis that distant prayer or the other alternative treatments had any impact on health outcomes. But curiously, in a June 29, 2004, *Washington Post* article on alternative medicine, Dr. Krucoff was quoted as reporting that in MANTRA II, "the combination of the bedside therapies and the prayer intervention creates a trend to improve survival." That is, he reported that the group of patients who received both prayer from the intercessors and the various other alternative treatments tended to do better than the patients receiving standard care alone, standard care plus prayer, or standard care plus the alternative treatments. *The Washington Post* article converted this "trend" to a statistically significant effect, further sustaining the myth about the healing power of prayer.

About a week later, on July 8, 2004, a press release from the Parliament of the World's Religions announced the establishment of the "Office of Prayer Research," whose aim was "to advance scientific research on the effects of prayer and to serve as a conduit for the exchange of information coming from the scores of prayer studies scientists conduct each year in the U.S. and throughout the world." According to this release, Dr. Krucoff was part of that announcement, which reported, "The MANTRA study revealed that of all patients tested, the lowest absolute patient complications were observed in patients assigned to offsite prayer. These results were significant enough to warrant further study."

Notice that this quote from a July 2004 press conference refers to one of the findings from the MANTRA pilot study published in 2001. The announcement is important for several reasons. It fails to report that "the lowest absolute level of complications" in favor of the prayer group was not a *significant* finding. More disingenuously, it fails to note that the negative findings of the more definitive MANTRA II study were already known and had been presented eight months earlier.

The myth continued its steady gallop. DukeMedNews, the Web site of the Duke University Medical Center, *currently* contains an October 31, 2001 news release about Krucoff's studies. It indicates that in the pilot study, patients receiving prayer "appeared to have better clinical outcomes" than a control group. Patients receiving any of the alternative treatments did 25 to 30 percent better than the control group. This report then adds that this study was too small for these findings to be statistically significant, so a larger study was launched. Even though the results were nonsignificant, DukeMedNews reports them anyway while failing to mention the inconvenient facts that in the pilot study all the deaths occurred in the noetic groups. It remains on the Web site despite the fact that the results of MANTRA II showing no effect of prayer or other alternative treatments have already been published.

From this we can see how gullible reporting combined with exaggerated or misleading statements can create a mythical medical treatment that can actually compromise real medical care: eight months or so *after* Krucoff presented the negative findings from MANTRA II, he remarked to *The Washington Post* that there was a trend toward better outcomes for these alternative treatments (from MANTRA II), and he told the assembled press at the Parliament of the World's Religions that the prayer group had the lowest absolute level of postintervention complications (from the MANTRA pilot study).

Apart from the obvious disingenuousness of failing to report that MANTRA II had shown no significant effects, there are other misleading but subtle aspects of these accounts. The first claim, from MANTRA II, that the combination of prayer and other alternative treatments had the best outcome, was about outcome defined as *death*. This is the "trend" toward better survival among the recipients of combined treatment. In the second claim, based on the MANTRA pilot study, researchers touted the impact of prayer on *patient complications*, a completely different outcome variable. To compare strictly, Krucoff should have referred to the pilot study findings about death. The problem is that in the pilot study, all the deaths occurred in the alternative conditions. And, of course, none of these pilot study findings was statistically significant. Krucoff failed to mention either of these facts.

These discrepancies may seem minor, but they raise concerns relevant to the sharpshooter's fallacy: that the researchers kept testing hypotheses until they found something that they deemed interesting. One time they tested death. Another time they tested outcomes during hospitalization. Sometimes they tested the combination of prayer and other treatments. Other times, they tested prayer and the alternative treatments separately. But, of course, none of these findings was significant.

MANTRA thus provides us with a wonderful example of one of the most worrisome practices in science: the release of scientific information through the popular press. It took almost two years after the presentation of the MANTRA II findings at the October 2003 conference for the findings to be published. During that time, media reports, encouraged by comments by Dr. Krucoff, suggested that the effects of prayer and the other alternative treatments had been demonstrated. The lesson: be careful about scientific information presented at press conferences, and about the gullible and poorly informed reporters who present them to the reading public.

## CONFLICTING FINDINGS: QUALITY OF PUBLICATION

Sometimes even published studies that use apparently acceptable research designs come to different conclusions. Since many reputable sources can come to different conclusions, we must ask, how can we determine which is the correct conclusion? Just because two competing claims come from *published* scientific articles does not make them equivalent in scientific value. One key indicator of the relative quality of scientific articles is the journals that publish them.

Simply put, some journals are better than others. Knowing whether reports are published in first-rate or lower-level journals can help us determine the value of these reports. Thanks to the Institute for Scientific Information (ISI), we can obtain some guidance on the relative quality of journals in many different fields of science. The ISI recognizes that one measure of the value of a scientific report is how often other scientists cite it. Papers that are considered high in quality are cited more frequently than those seen as lower in quality. Correspondingly, journals that publish papers that are cited often are stronger than journals that publish papers cited only infrequently. Thus, one index of the strength or weakness of any particular scientific journal is how often the papers it publishes are cited by other researchers. The ISI refers to this index as the "impact factor" of a journal, and information on the impact factor is contained in the ISI's Science Citation Index, available at most libraries and on the Internet.

According to the Science Citation Index, within the field of general medicine (as opposed to medical specialties such as cardiology and oncology), the three most prestigious journals are the *The New England Journal of Medicine,* the *Journal of the American Medical Association* (*JAMA*), and *The Lancet.* Their impact factors are 38.570, 24.831, and 21.713 respectively. Here are the top fifteen journals within the field of general medicine in 2004. They are listed in order of their rank, along with the impact factor.

| | |
|---|---|
| 1. *New England Journal of Medicine* | 38.570 |
| 2. *Journal of the American Medical Association* | 24.831 |
| 3. *Lancet* | 21.713 |
| 4. *Annals of Internal Medicine* | 13.114 |
| 5. *Annual Review of Medicine* | 11.200 |
| 6. *Archives of Internal Medicine* | 7.508 |
| 7. *British Medical Journal* | 7.038 |
| 8. *Canadian Medical Association* | 5.941 |
| 9. *American Journal of Medicine* | 4.179 |
| 10. *Mayo Clinic Proceedings* | 3.746 |
| 11. *Medicine* | 3.727 |
| 12. *Annals of Medicine* | 3.617 |
| 13. *Journal of Internal Medicine* | 3.590 |
| 14. *American Journal of Preventive Medicine* | 3.188 |
| 15. *Current Medical Research and Opinion* | 2.928 |

We can use the ISI's impact factor to get a sense of the level of the journals in which studies of religion and health are published. To do this, let's examine the quality of the journals cited in a review of religion and health that was published in a peer-reviewed journal. In 2003, Lynda Powell from Rush-Presbyterian Medical Center in Chicago and two colleagues published what is arguably the strongest review in this field. We'll examine it in detail later in the book, but for now, to get a sense of the quality of the publications that appear in the literature on religion and health, we'll compute the average impact factor for the articles cited in this review.

For comparison purposes, we can do the same thing with studies that evaluate the relationship between depression and heart disease, taken from a recent review of this topic by Robert Carney and others. I've selected this second review because it represents another hot area in behavioral medicine, as well as being a review of articles that look at connections between health and a person's psychological makeup. Depression is a psychological characteristic that appears to influence physical health, just as religious involvement, another psychological characteristic, is thought to influence physical health.

If we look carefully at the different impact factors, interesting patterns emerge. The review paper on depression and heart disease identifies 17 studies that address this matter. The average impact factor of the journals in which these studies appear is 9.65. In contrast, the Powell paper that looks at the connections between religion and health reviews 112 papers, and the average impact factor for all those journals that the ISI rates was 4.71. Part of the reason for this substantial difference is that Carney et al. were much more selective than Powell and colleagues. By being more selective, they excluded poor-quality studies.

But that, of course, is precisely the point. Reviews of studies of religion and health have to rely on poor-quality studies because without them, there would be very few studies to review. Thus, by objective standards established by the Institute for Scientific Information, the journals in which studies of religion and health appear are of far lower scientific prestige than the journals in which studies of depression and heart disease appear. This difference would be even greater if the Powell paper had not included citations from top journals like *The Lancet* and *The New England Journal of Medicine*. The interesting thing about the papers cited from these prestigious journals is that they either have nothing to do with religion and health or are articles critical of the proposed connection.

So one guide for anyone interested in determining the value of scientific information on religion and health is to consider where a paper was published. While it is not a hard and fast rule, papers published in *The New England Journal of Medicine* generally are regarded as better science than those published in, for example, *The International Journal of Psychiatry in Medicine* (*IJPM*), rated by the ISI as the seventy-seventh most important journal in psychiatry in 2004. The *IJPM* is a favorite outlet for studies on religion and health. It is fair to assume that papers published in the *IJPM* are of lower quality than those published in *The New England Journal of Medicine*, although there may be exceptions.

## PRIMARY OR SECONDARY SOURCE?

Significant discoveries in medicine are published in the kind of journals described above. The reports of these findings are called *primary sources* because the scientists who actually conducted the research write them. But in medicine and in other fields of science, the amount of information published every year is so enormous that it is difficult for all but the most dedicated readers to keep up with each and every study. For this reason, a great many readers rely on *secondary sources,* reviews of the original primary scientific articles. Like primary reports of findings, secondary sources may appear in journals that vary widely in quality. Often books function as secondary sources too, reviewing a great many research studies.

Secondary sources serve a useful function in summarizing a large literature. They provide readers with considerable information in a relatively brief time that otherwise might require a great many more hours to acquire. In this sense, secondary sources are highly efficient. But secondary sources have a great disadvantage, too: they represent the views of the authors of the review, not necessarily of the writers of the scientific articles reviewed. Because secondary sources attempt to summarize the findings of many original articles, they include only some of the material from the original articles while excluding other information. This other information, unfortunately, may be important.

Some secondary sources are excellent references. The two cited above, by Powell and colleagues and by Carney and colleagues, are examples of high-quality secondary sources. But some secondary sources are particularly misleading about the research findings. Let's look at a few examples:

In a review paper, Dr. Paul Mueller and his colleagues at the Mayo Clinic reported that "at least 18 prospective studies have shown that religiously involved persons live longer." We don't even have to look at these studies too closely to see that such a conclusion is, at best, an uncritical one. Three are from Comstock's studies, which we saw were compromised by the failure to control for the confounding factors that were likely to eliminate the significant finding. Three others were from the same set of data, the Alameda County Study. These studies were connected, and to report them as independent is misleading. Further compromising the conclusion, only women and not men were the beneficiaries of religious involvement in the Alameda County data. The latter is true of several other studies Mueller et al. cite. One study that supposedly showed a connection between religious involvement and mortality in fact did not show this effect. It showed that social activities (which included church attendance along with going to movies, playing cards, etc.) and productive activities (gardening, preparing meals, shopping) were associated with reduced mortality, but it didn't show a relationship between religious involvement and mortality. Mueller and his colleagues concluded this section by citing the findings from a review paper without giving due consideration to confounding factors. If you read that review paper yourself, you discover that after control for clinical measures of health, risk behaviors like smoking and obesity, and social support and other social factors, the relationship between religious involvement and mortality was no longer significant. Given all of this, for Mueller and his colleagues to claim that eighteen studies have shown that the religiously involved live longer is a gross exaggeration. This typifies the problem with secondary studies. When reviewing studies for such an article, the authors writing the review can interpret the data in any way they choose, sometimes with little regard for the actual findings reported in the original papers.

Let's look at another review paper touting the health effects of religion. Drs. Jeffrey Levin and Harold Vanderpool looked at the relationship between religion and blood pressure. Levin is properly regarded as the founder of what has come to be called the "epidemiology of religion," the study of religion and health. Like the Mueller article, this one is full of exaggeration and misinterpretation. Levin and Vanderpool may think that they've demonstrated that lack of religious involvement is associated with elevated blood pressure, but in fact the only thing they've shown is that if you take science seriously, reading this misleading article can raise your blood pressure.

Levin and Vanderpool conclude that "the characteristics and functions of religion have salutary effects on blood pressure." Among the evidence they use to bolster this statement is a 1963 paper by Norman Scotch that reports a protective effect of religious attendance and church membership, i.e., those who attend church and are church members have lower blood pressure than those who don't. This paper, like so many others in this tradition, illustrates what some have referred to, rather poetically, as "data dredging."

Data dredging refers to the practice of fishing through large data sets until you come up with something that appears to be statistically significant. In other words, researchers intent upon finding a result will look and look and look until they identify something they can report. This can happen with analysis of your own data (we've already reviewed examples of this). It can also be seen in secondary sources. In this case, the data dredging was accomplished by Levin and Vanderpool as secondary reviewers. If you read the paper by Scotch, you recognize immediately that the original paper had nothing to do with the protective effects of religious commitment, as they imply. It was about the impact of assimilation into new societies, either by immigration or moving from rural to urban life; religious affiliation was used merely as an index of assimilation into the new society. That is, joining a church or other religious institution was used by Scotch as an indicator that the immigrants had become assimilated. The differences in blood pressure identified by Levin and Vanderpool represent only one of many different comparisons that Scotch made in his original paper, raising the problem of multiple comparisons we reviewed above. But because Scotch was not principally concerned with the health benefits of religious activities, there was no reason for him to be concerned with multiple comparisons. On the other hand, reviewers using these studies to claim associations between religious involvement and health have a different obligation. If they dredge the findings of a study to pick out the one or two statistics that support their views, they must address this methodological problem.

Let us delve a little further into Levin and Vanderpool's study to see how authors of secondary reviews can present the material in an original paper to suit their own needs. One paper they consider supportive of the proposition that religious commitment protects against high blood pressure, by Yechiel Friedlander and Jeremy Kark, demonstrated that Israeli women whose fathers had five or more years of yeshiva education had lower diastolic blood pressure than women whose fathers had less religious education. Often, to understand how misleading secondary sources are, you have to read the original papers carefully to learn what has artfully been omitted from the review article. In this case, however, the flaw is right in front of us. We have no idea whatsoever about the religious commitment of the women whose blood pressure was measured. Levin and Vanderpool are making the unstated, and therefore unquestioned, assumption that the women whose fathers had more yeshiva education are more committed to Judaism than those whose fathers had spent less time in a yeshiva. They make no allowances for the possibility that the fathers might ultimately have rejected Judaism or that the daughters might have done the same. We know about the fathers' degree of commitment only in terms of the years spent in the yeshiva. Considering these possibilities, how is it possible to conclude, as Levin and Vanderpool have, that there is a protective effect of religious commitment here? It's not possible, and the other studies reviewed in this paper are no more supportive of a protective effect of religious commitment.

In general, other secondary sources of the literature on religion and health are no less uncritical and misleading. Secondary sources serve an important function in science. They synthesize a large literature, making it accessible to those who don't have the time to read all the papers they summarize. But secondary sources vary enormously in quality, and with the exception of the Powell review discussed above, most are inaccurate in their treatment of the religion-health literature.

## EXTREME CLAIMS

Another aspect of questionable scientific findings that can alert you to bad research is the extreme nature of claims that some researchers make about their work. This is especially true in the case of claims about the effects of distant intercessory prayer (IP). Adherents of IP claim that the healing intentions or prayers of some people influence the health of other people and that this effect operates over great distances. IP researchers embellish their published work with allusions to scientific breakthroughs of the past. Dr. Larry Dossey, for example, quotes Sir John Maddox, the former editor of the prestigious journal *Nature*: "The most important discoveries of the next 50 years are likely to be the ones of which we cannot now even conceive." The implication is clear: studies of IP are truly revolutionary, but because modern scientists are too narrow-minded, they cannot see this.

We'll review the studies of intercessory prayer in Chapter 9, but extreme claims can be found for other areas of research in the religion-and-health field. For example, physicians David Larson and Dale Matthews argue for spiritual and religious interventions in medical practice and boldly call for the "wall of separation" between medicine and religion to be torn down. Clearly, they see themselves as scientific revolutionaries breaking down the resistance of the old guard. Matthews, as we've already seen, has gone so far as to assert that "the medicine of the future is going to be prayer and Prozac." "Do religious beliefs and activities really keep one mentally or physically healthier and reduce mortality, as some claim? If so, this finding has major implications for our struggling health care system." This statement from Koenig, McCullough, and Larson suggests that the incorporation of religious practices into clinical medicine in the U.S. will transform the field. Hyperbole abounds when researchers don't want people thinking too deeply about their work or looking too closely at their results. At this point, we should remember the words of L. Frank Baum's Wizard of Oz as he tries to dissuade the visitors from looking beyond the smoke and mirrors: "Pay no attention to the man behind the curtain."

Others also make extreme, even grandiose statements about what's best for the practice of medicine. "I believe the practice of basic spiritual skills is just too important to be left solely to pastoral professionals," says Dr. Walter Larimore, implying grandly that physicians should be involved in the spiritual lives of their patients. Quoting Arthur Kornhaber, Larimore suggests that excluding religion and spirituality from clinical consultations is malpractice: "'To exclude God from a consultation is a form of malpractice. Spirituality is wonder, joy and shouldn't be left in the clinical closet.' Let's don't!"

"This is no routine paper," Harvard physician Herbert Benson said rather grandiosely, explaining why his paper on the effect of distant prayer on outcomes after heart surgery had still not been published more than three years after data collection ended. "What you're looking at obviously is not a typical intervention, not at all. We are at the interface of science and religion here, and there are boundary issues that you would not have for almost any other paper." My personal favorite is from Matthews, Larson, and Constance Barry, who put a spin on their data that would satisfy health insurance providers the world over and give it the gloss of the hard-nosed businessman: "In this era of cost containment, prayer may be a particularly cost-effective as well as efficacious form of treatment." Imagine that: we can save money by implementing distant prayer as part of our medical care system. Well, they must be right! After all, they're doctors.

Contrast these boastful statements with the remarks of a truly revolutionary scientist, physicist Richard Feynman, who won the 1965 Nobel Prize in Physics for his work in quantum electrodynamics. In his lecture to the Swedish Academy of Science, a customary part of the award ceremony, he was exceedingly modest, declaring "what a stupid fellow" he had been early in his career and readily acknowledging how his infatuation with an idea that turned out to be wrong had led him to ignore its many problems. He went on to admit that he did not understand some important elements of quantum mechanics and that he spent almost as much time on unsuccessful matters as he spent on ones that ultimately succeeded. Feynman did not say anything like "this is no routine paper" or that his discovery "had major implications" for physics. He did not declare that his work would transform the field. He allowed his work to speak for itself, and clearly, it did. No overstatement was necessary.

So where does this leave us? In this chapter, we have identified several other key features to consider when evaluating claims that religious activity and involvement are associated with beneficial health outcomes. Let's make a quick review:

- Only reports that appear in peer-reviewed journals should be considered as valid, and even these may vary in quality. Those made in books and magazine articles or in the print or broadcast media should be regarded with caution or even with suspicion.

- The most solid claims will be published in the highest-quality medical journals like the *New England Journal of Medicine, JAMA,* and *Lancet* or in outstanding general-science journals like *Science* or *Nature.* Reports of findings that appear in lower-level journals, for example in the *International Journal of Psychiatry and Medicine,* should be viewed with greater skepticism.

- Claims based on presentations at scientific meetings or made in press conferences should be considered as fact only if they have been accompanied or followed by reports of these claims made in peer-reviewed journals.

- Statements about evidence of connections between religion and health made in secondary sources should never be accepted unless you have actually read the primary sources yourself. Remember that these secondary sources, especially those in book form, more often reflect the perspective of the reviewer than of the authors of the studies reviewed.

- Beware of scientific information presented at press conferences or briefings unless they accompany the publication of a research paper. Without an actual published study, we can't be sure that what is reported at the conference is really reflected in the research.

- Finally, be especially cautious about bold claims, especially those about revolutionary science. Scientific revolutions do occur, but they are *very* uncommon. When they do take place, they are based on organized theories that permit specific, testable predictions about phenomena that were previously inexplicable. That's what makes them revolutionary. By this standard, nothing in the field of religion and health is revolutionary science.

# IS THERE REALLY A HEALTH ADVANTAGE
# TO BEING RELIGIOUSLY ACTIVE?

Ideally, to determine whether there really is a health advantage to being religiously active, we'd examine all of the studies that truly are relevant to the supposed health benefits of religious involvement. We have neither the time nor the space for this. So instead, let's select for examination reports that *others* believe make the strongest case for this effect by examining the scientific articles cited in two reviews of the medical literature on the benefits of religious activities and practices on cardiovascular health. One review examining twelve studies was published in the *Journal of Cardiopulmonary Rehabilitation*. The other is the voluminous *Handbook of Religion and Health* by Koenig and colleagues. For the *Handbook*, which stretches to more than seven hundred pages, we restrict our review to the chapters on heart disease and hypertension, which examined eighty-nine studies in total.

The studies in these two reviews are what the authors believe represent the *strongest* evidence demonstrating the cardiovascular-health-enhancing value of religious activities. Frederic Luskin's review, for example, reports that "evidence continues to mount that demonstrates the positive value of spiritual and religious factors in maintaining health." Koenig et al. report that "of the 16 studies that have examined the relationship between level of religious involvement and blood pressure, 14 (88 percent) found lower blood pressure among the more religious." Presumably, then, these studies are solid.

To make his claim of mounting evidence, Luskin reviews twelve scientific papers on cardiovascular disease. Let's ask ourselves an initial, important question: How many of these twelve papers were actually relevant to the health benefits of religious practices? After we answer that question, let's proceed to another: Of these, how many are methodologically sound enough to permit us to draw solid conclusions that there is a health benefit to religious involvement? Of the twelve papers, one was a review of other studies. Two additional papers were about denominational differences and health. A fourth paper was published only as an abstract—a summary of the research itself and not the complete report. As such, it didn't contain enough information for an adequate evaluation. Therefore, of the twelve papers, four could not provide information on the health benefits of religious practices. What can we say about the remaining eight?

Two more papers failed to control for multiple comparisons, a problem we already talked about. In fact, we've already examined one of these: Koenig's study of attendance and blood pressure in which at least 126 statistical tests were conducted with no control whatsoever for multiple comparisons but that nevertheless reported some "statistically significant" findings. Two of the six remaining studies were about the benefits of organized religious activity on blood pressure. Both used the same set of data but came to different conclusions. One found that subjects who reported high levels of religious attendance and felt that religion was important had lower diastolic (but not systolic) blood pressure when they were compared to subjects reporting low levels of attendance and a low degree of importance of religion. The other study, which used the same set of data, reported that the frequency of church attendance was positively related to systolic (but not diastolic) blood pressure. These studies illustrate how, using precisely the same data, you can get completely different findings depending upon how you analyze the data. One group found that religious attendance was associated with lower diastolic blood pressure but not systolic blood pressure. Another found an effect on systolic blood pressure but no difference in diastolic blood pressure. These findings cannot both be correct; moreover, neither of these studies controlled for the factor most closely related to church attendance: the health status of the participants. As we saw above, if you are already sick, you are more likely to have high blood pressure, more likely to die, and less likely to be able to attend church. That leaves four. What about them?

One, a study of patients admitted for coronary artery bypass surgery, found that those rating themselves as moderately to highly religious had significantly shorter lengths of stay in the hospital. But like so many studies in this area, no analysis of the effects of confounders such as other health indicators like blood pressure, social variables like marital status, or health behaviors like smoking was conducted. Therefore, we don't know if these findings were really the product of other factors. Another study also examined bypass surgery patients. In an appropriately conducted analysis, one item ("strength or comfort from religion") from a five-item scale of religiosity was found to be associated with mortality independent of history of cardiac surgery, functional status, age, and a measure of social participation. That is, even after considering these potentially confounding factors, the association between "comfort from religion" and reduced mortality remained. The problem is that none of the other items of this scale, for example, the ubiquitous attendance at religious services or religious social contact, or the composite score itself, which was computed by summing the scores from each item (all of which have been used in many other studies), was related to mortality. In this study, as in so many others, the failure to control for multiple comparisons arises. Why should we focus solely on "comfort from religion" but not on these other variables?

Two studies are left. What about them?

The two remaining studies cited by Luskin also have serious methodological problems. One suggested health benefits of religious involvement to heart transplant patients, but again, this finding was the result of one of forty-two statistical tests with no control for multiple comparisons. The final paper of the twelve suggested, according to Luskin, that religious coping was protective, but in fact there is nothing whatsoever about protection in this paper. That makes a group of twelve papers in which not a single one is adequate to demonstrate an advantage to the more religiously involved. However, that didn't stop Luskin from making claims about the "mounting evidence," something that should have given us pause in the first place. We saw above how misleading secondary sources can be. Luskin's paper provides us with a superb example, and it also permits us to see what a researcher who aims to prove a connection between religion and good health regards as the best studies in the field. Clearly, they barely make the cut.

## HANDBOOK OF RELIGION AND HEALTH

Let's now turn to Koenig's *Handbook*. This is a long book, ponderous in appearance and purporting to be the last word, or many last words, on the subject of religion and health. Its heft and publisher of origin are both meant to command respect. Published by the eminent academic publisher Oxford University Press, the book weighs in at three and a half pounds and extends to some seven hundred plus pages. It is a weighty tome, but we will deal here with only two chapters. I'll summarize them for you, but anyone interested in reading a detailed analysis of the eighty-nine scientific reports on cardiovascular health cited by Koenig et al. in the *Handbook* can read Emilia Bagiella's and my paper on this topic. As a whole, the book is filled with research studies that have serious methodological problems, and to make matters worse, many of the findings are simply misrepresented.

Of the eighty-nine studies we'll consider, thirty-three were studies of denominational differences in health. This means that the studies contrasted the health of different religious denominations. For example, a study might have compared levels of cholesterol in Baptists and Lutherans. Demonstrating denominational differences may be of interest, but these studies don't tell us anything about the putative health benefits of religious involvement. They tell us nothing about how praying or reading the Bible affects liver disease or cataracts. An additional eleven were reviews of other studies, case reports, or mere descriptions of projects. Three were published only in abstract form and cannot be critically reviewed because abstracts lack essential detail. By the criteria of the *Handbook* itself, eight additional studies showed no association between religious activity and health. This leaves only thirty-four of the original eighty-nine papers (38 percent) that can be the basis of claims about the direction and strength of the religion-health relationship. After reviewing these thirty-four, we found that thirty of them contained serious methodological flaws or were so misinterpreted or misrepresented that they cannot possibly be used as evidence for an effect of religion on health. Let's look at a few of these thirty-four studies.

## Studies with Methodological Problems

The *Handbook* identifies a paper by Jane Leserman et al. as one that demonstrates a positive effect of religion on cardiovascular disease by reporting the results of a small trial of relaxation on cardiac surgery patients. Leserman and colleagues reported that cardiac arrhythmias in the immediate postoperative period were lower in the group that received relaxation training than in the control group. However, this was the only difference between the groups. They did not differ in the other seven variables collected, including blood pressure, pain, or postoperative hospital stay. Here we have yet another example of the sharpshooter's fallacy: collecting a great many outcome variables and seeing if any turn out to be related to the intervention. If the authors had *predicted in advance* that the relaxation training would influence cardiac arrhythmias and none of the other variables, then we'd really have a finding of importance. But at least as reported in the paper, there's no reason the difference should have been in arrhythmias rather than blood pressure or pain or postoperative stay. The authors of the paper acknowledge that this one significant finding may be the result of chance alone, considering that they collected so many other variables that failed to achieve significance. Koenig and colleagues, however, do not.

Several of the papers the *Handbook* regards as positive fail to control for confounding. Its treatment of the study by Ratree Sudsaung et al. is especially enlightening. The *Handbook* reports that in this study, fifty-two male college students were taught Buddhist meditation and were compared to thirty control students who were not. Meditation subjects but not the controls had lower blood pressure at three- and six-week follow-up compared to their levels at study entry. What the original paper makes clear, however, but the *Handbook* does not, is that the groups were not randomly assigned. Rather, they were self-selected, with meditation subjects volunteering to be cloistered as monks for two months during their summer vacation, during which they engaged in no activities other than "walking about 1 km to receive food from people in the morning." Control subjects stayed at home for summer vacation.

The problems with this study are painfully obvious. First, subjects were not randomly assigned to receive meditation. Rather, the treatment subjects self-selected to be cloistered for two months. By definition, people who choose to spend their summers cloistered in a monastery are different from people who choose to spend their summers in conventional ways. We don't know for certain what those differences might be, but we can guess. Perhaps they were better off economically (they didn't need to work for the summer as most college students do). Perhaps they were concerned about their stressful lives and saw the study as an opportunity to relax. Second, the treatment subjects differed from the control subjects in one other highly significant way: they lived for two months in a cloister, protected from the stress of the outside world. This alone could have accounted for the blood pressure differences between the groups. If we took any of us, cloistered us in a monastery for two months, and had us read, or listen to music, or even knit sweaters, our blood pressure would almost certainly go down. This effect has nothing to do with religion.

Two other papers had inadequate or nonexistent control groups. Michael Cooper and Maurice Aygen reported on the effect on blood lipids of transcendental meditation (TM), a technique of meditation based on Hindu tradition that promotes deep relaxation through the use of a mantra. The number of subjects was small (twelve in the treatment group and eleven in the control group), and assignment to treatment condition was not random. Treatment subjects volunteered to participate in the study while attending lectures on TM. Control subjects were recruited from a medical outpatient clinic. Four of the subjects originally in the treatment group deemed insufficiently active in meditation were reassigned to the control group, a flagrant violation of scientific standards. Only the intervention subjects showed a significant decline in blood cholesterol. Another study, by Barry Blackwell et al., also had no control group.

In another study identified by the *Handbook* as showing a relationship between religious involvement and cardiovascular health, Stig Wenneberg et al. examined the impact of TM on reactivity to laboratory stressors (mental arithmetic and public speaking). Reactivity refers to the increase in a physiological variable, e.g., heart rate or blood pressure, in response to a stressor. Scientists are interested in reactivity because some evidence suggests that repeated increases in heart rate or blood pressure are part of the disease process in heart disease. Ambulatory blood pressure (ABP) also was examined.

In this clinical trial, while subjects were randomly assigned to a TM or health education condition, there was substantial dropout. Among those who remained in the study, no differences were found between pretreatment and posttreatment reactivity to laboratory stressors. Similarly, there were no treatment differences in ABP when all subjects were considered. When only high-compliance subjects (in both conditions) were examined, the TM subjects actually had higher systolic blood pressure (SBP) reactivity to the preparation for the speech task and to the speech task itself. That is, the TM subjects did *worse* than the control subjects. But high compliers in the TM group had lower posttreatment ambulatory diastolic blood pressure than control subjects. At best, this study is equivocal with respect to an advantage to the TM group.

Finally, the *Handbook* identifies as positive a study by Miller on the impact of remote healing. This paper is so bad that it would be funny if it wasn't considered by Koenig and colleagues to provide evidence of a health benefit of religion. The study reported that hypertensive patients who were the recipients of "remote healing" had a greater reduction in SBP than those in the control group. No information about the patients, except that there were ninety-six of them, was presented. There were eight "healers": four were "Science of Mind Practitioners," one was a Presbyterian minister, another was a Church of Christ minister, one was the "Director of the Seventh Sense Institute," and the final healer was simply "a gifted individual whose healing abilities have been verified by both doctors and scientists." Healer Mr. B.B., we are told in the paper, described his procedure as "Televisual Healing." He uses this procedure to "contact the inner mind of the subject and observe the true nature of the injury or malfunction" and then uses "mental pictures to show the subject's inner mind how to correct this." I am not making this up.

Apart from this nonsense, it is unclear how long the interval between pre- and post-intervention data collection was. Moreover, the SBP finding was the only one that achieved statistical significance (diastolic blood pressure, pulse rate, weight, and health status [a poorly defined composite measure] did not change). In addition, data were presented only for the patients of four of the healers "who had the highest number of returned patients." Assuming that "returned patients" means patients who did not drop out, this means that statistical analysis was conducted on an incomplete data set.

These all are studies that according to the *Handbook* qualify as showing a favorable effect of religious involvement on cardiovascular outcomes. Can Koenig and colleagues seriously expect us to believe that these studies constitute solid evidence of a beneficial effect on health? It is often said that success has many fathers, but failure is an orphan. In this case, it's failure that has many fathers. It's hard to know who is more to blame for these weak studies. In some cases, it's the researchers themselves. In other cases, it's the journals for accepting them for publication. But at least in some cases, the authors (and by implication, the journals) have acknowledged the limitations of their research. For example, Leserman and colleagues recognized that because they collected data on so many outcome variables, their one significant finding might really be a chance occurrence. The real responsibility lies with the authors of the *Handbook,* who cite these studies as supporting their claim of health benefits of religious involvement without qualification, when in fact they provide no support whatsoever. But it gets worse.

## Misrepresentations in the *Handbook*

The studies discussed above were selected because, presumably, they represent the most persuasive cases for an effect of religious involvement on health. Nevertheless, they all had methodological problems so serious that we can't draw any conclusions from them. In this section, let's examine some studies, also thought to demonstrate the health benefits of religious involvement, that don't really have any of these methodological problems. These studies, however, have problems of a different sort and represent another problematic element of Koenig's *Handbook.* Rather than being flawed because of methodological problems, many of the studies in the *Handbook* are simply misrepresented in a way that furthers the illusion of a connection between religious practice and good health.

One of my favorite examples of misrepresentation of scientific evidence in the *Handbook* is a paper about a weight-control program. In the view of the *Handbook,* this paper qualifies as a study of religion and health simply because it was conducted in a church. The program itself had nothing to do with religion. It was a standard, behaviorally oriented weight-control program. According to the authors, it employed "techniques commonly used in behavioral modification programs." These techniques included self-monitoring of food intake, goal setting, social support, and exercise. The program had limited success: after eight weeks, subjects lost an average of six pounds and lowered their blood pressure. By the standards of the *Handbook,* if the program was held in a gym it would have been a sports-related weight-control program. Or if it had been held at Merrill Lynch, it would have been a financial weight-control program. The venue had nothing to do with what kind of a program it was. To call it a religious intervention is silly and misleading.

Other studies also were seriously misrepresented. Three studies, while about religious activities, are cited as positive when in fact they report no significant effects. The first, by Karen Hixson et al., is cited as a study with one or more positive associations between a religious variable and a health outcome. In this study of religious commitment, health behaviors, and blood pressure, data were obtained on 112 women. There is not a single statistically significant finding in the entire paper. In fact, the authors themselves report that the results of the analyses they conducted examining the influence of religiosity on blood pressure for all subjects did not reveal any statistically significant findings. The second paper, by Koenig himself, along with some of his colleagues, is cited in the chapter summary as marginally positive. It is true that among the twenty-six primary statistical tests reported in this paper, eight were at least marginally significant, but for three of them, the findings were in the *opposite* of the predicted direction. For example, private religious behaviors like reading the Bible or private prayer were more common among people in poorer health than among those in excellent health. The third study, also reported as positive, examined differences in health among Rhode Island residents who either were church members or were not. There appeared to be an advantage among church members in smoking and in diastolic (but not systolic) blood pressure, but church members were likely to weigh more. Koenig et al. represent this study as one demonstrating a health advantage to the religiously active, but according to the authors of the study itself, "overall, we found that church members were not different from non-members with respect to most CVD risk factors. With the exception of cigarette-smoking status, majority-church members may actually have more adverse CVD-risk-factor profiles."

The authors of the *Handbook* believe, as do many others, that their massive work represents the definitive examination of the literature on religion and health, assembling a compendium of research studies that most strongly demonstrate the health benefits of religious involvement. The best way to appreciate this effort is to compare it to the work of a historically significant but now obscure psychologist. At the turn of the twentieth century, American psychology was dominated by Edward Bradford Titchener of Cornell University. The details of his work are unimportant for our purposes, but the approach he took, one of extraordinary thoroughness and voluminous research, is in some ways reminiscent of the *Handbook*. Titchener's psychology disappeared from the face of the earth precisely because in his thoroughness, he ended up demonstrating how completely wrong it was. For this reason, Edna Heidbreder, the great historian of psychology, described his work as "a gallant and enlightening failure." Ironically, the great strength of the *Handbook* is also its downfall: because of their thoroughness, Koenig and colleagues have assembled the most comprehensive list of research studies thought to prove the health benefits of religious activity. What they have done instead is to show us definitively how incredibly weak the evidence actually is. The *Handbook* may not be gallant, but it certainly is enlightening.

The Latin expression *caveat emptor* means "let the buyer beware." It applies perfectly to the questionable evaluations of the evidence about the health benefits of religious involvement. At least in the case of cardiovascular disease, the studies provide no basis for claims of a health advantage to the religiously active. Virtually all the studies that these reviewers claimed show health benefits of religious involvement are flawed or seriously misrepresented. Remember the cautionary tale from the previous chapter: *Be extremely careful when reading secondary sources.*

This examination was restricted to studies of cardiovascular health, and although the very same problems are likely to afflict studies of religious involvement and other health outcomes, we are reluctant to draw firm conclusions about them. Fortunately, however, another group of researchers has done this for us. Earlier, we considered a study by Dr. Lynda Powell and colleagues that systematically reviewed the entire literature on religious involvement and physical health outcomes, not just those relating to cardiovascular disease. In this review, the authors examined the evidence relevant to nine different hypotheses about the health benefits of religious involvement.

Before we go any further, you should ask yourselves, why consider this review of the literature? After all, we've just discussed how misleading some reviews can be. Why trust this one? This is absolutely the right question to ask, and part of the answer is that the journal in which this review was published, the *American Psychologist*, is the flagship journal of the American Psychological Association and one of the most prestigious journals in the field. Because of its strength, we can have more confidence in papers that appear in it.

Moreover, the methodology employed by Powell and colleagues is greatly superior to the uncritical methods we've seen in other reviews. Unlike these other reviewers, Powell and colleagues eliminated studies that failed to control for potential confounders. Because they were concerned about whether religious variables influenced physical health, they eliminated cross-sectional studies. We saw above that these studies cannot shed light on causality.

In addition, their review excluded studies that inadequately measured religious or spiritual variables and physical health outcomes. They also disregarded studies that did not present statistical analyses. Finally, they did not include studies that came from the same set of research subjects. This distinguishes the Powell review from the review by Mueller and colleagues, discussed above, that identified eighteen studies demonstrating an effect of religious involvement on mortality.

Powell and colleagues looked at studies that shed light on nine different hypotheses about religion and health. The table below lists these hypotheses and the conclusions Powell and colleagues drew. Evidence was considered "persuasive" if there were at least three supportive studies without any significant methodological flaws or five studies that were at least generally sound. A hypothesis was considered to have "some" support if there was one supportive study with no flaws or at least two that were generally sound. Evidence was considered "inadequate" if the research base was too small to draw firm conclusions. Hypotheses were deemed "consistent failures" when studies repeatedly failed to support them. The methodological flaws Powell and colleagues considered should be familiar by now: control for confounders, imprecise measurement, control for multiple comparisons, and focusing narrowly on a finding in a single subgroup among others.

| HYPOTHESES | STRENGTH OF EVIDENCE |
|---|---|
| 1. Church/service attendance protects against death. | Persuasive |
| 2. Religion or spirituality protects against cardiovascular disease. | Some |
| 3. Religion or spirituality protects against cancer mortality. | Inadequate |
| 4. Deeply religious people are protected against death. | Consistent failures |
| 5. Religion or spirituality protects against disability. | Consistent failures |
| 6. Religion or spirituality slows the progression of cancer. | Consistent failures |
| 7. People who use religion to cope with difficulties live longer. | Inadequate |
| 8. Religion or spirituality improves recovery from acute illness. | Consistent failures |
| Religion or spirituality impedes recovery from acute illness. | Some |
| 9. Being prayed for improves physical recovery from acute illness. | Some |

As you can see from this table, while the nine hypotheses differed considerably, only in one case was the evidence supportive of an association between religious involvement and better health: Powell et al. reviewed eleven different studies that examined the association between attendance at religious services and mortality, and they concluded that the evidence was persuasive. People who reported that they attended religious services regularly had lower mortality than those attending services less frequently.

We'll come back to the attendance-mortality hypothesis in the next chapter to consider it more broadly, but let's look at some of the other hypotheses before we finish thinking about Powell's study. These researchers found only some evidence for the hypothesis that religion or spirituality protects against heart disease and even less evidence that it protects against cancer mortality. Evidence of protection against death, disability, or the progression of cancer consistently failed to support these hypotheses. With the exception of the attendance-mortality studies, the evidence of a health benefit of religious involvement was, in the view of Powell and colleagues, weak at best. Because the methods of this review and the stature of the journal in which it was published give us more confidence in its conclusions, we should examine the data in the one area that Powell and colleagues considered solid: the relationship between attendance at religious services and mortality.

# 8

## ATTENDANCE AT SERVICES AND MORTALITY

## DOES ATTENDANCE AT RELIGIOUS SERVICES AFFECT MORTALITY?

In one of the studies reviewed by Lynda Powell, by Robert Hummer and colleagues, 21,204 participants were interviewed about a wide range of topics, including their health and their religious practices. The data for the study were collected using an interview format. Individuals were asked, for example, how frequently they attended religious services. Did they attend more than once each week? Did they attend only once each week or once each month?

The entire group of more than 21,000 participants was followed for eight years. During this time, 2,016 participants from the original sample had died. Because information on attendance at religious services was collected during the first wave of data collection, the researchers could examine whether it was associated with mortality at follow-up. In fact, the researchers found that there was a link. Hummer and colleagues reported that increasing levels of self-reported attendance at religious services was associated with reduced likelihood of death eight years later. Several other longitudinal studies of large samples of participants also showed similar results. So Powell and colleagues, whose review we considered in the last chapter, were correct: studies looking at the link between attendance at religious services and mortality are the strongest studies in the field.

Despite these supportive studies, the association between attendance at religious services and mortality is problematic for several reasons:

- The link between attendance at religious services and mortality is an *association* that may not be causal. Just because there seems to be a link doesn't mean that one actually exists between two such seemingly disparate variables.
- Methodological problems in measuring attendance exist. We know that in research studies that use interview methods of data collection, respondents tend to shape their answers in ways they think will please the interviewer rather than respond with complete accuracy.
- The meaning of attendance, even if accurately measured, is open to interpretation. Because people go to religious services for a great many reasons, attendance does not always signify religious devotion. Does "attendance" merely mean that there is a warm body in a pew, or does it mean that someone is there, faithfully engaging fully in the service?
- The implications for medical practice of a connection between religious attendance and mortality, even if it is a causal connection, are far from clear. Therefore, physicians should not be putting together treatment plans that encourage patients to attend religious services regularly.

Let's now look closely at each of these problems.

# The Connection Between Religious Attendance and Mortality Is an Association That May Not Be Causal

The classic way of establishing causality in science is to conduct an experiment in which a sample of subjects is selected. One part of the sample is assigned, at random, to a treatment group. Another part is assigned to a control group. Whatever treatment is being studied is under the control of the experimenter and is administered to the treatment group but not the control group. The two groups are then evaluated to determine if they differ with respect to a primary variable. That variable is an outcome that is determined before the research gets under way. If, under these stringent conditions, the two groups differ, we can be reasonably certain that the difference is caused by the treatment. Our certainty derives from the fact that because of random assignment, we expect that, save for the treatment group's receiving the treatment agent, the two groups will not differ in any important respect from each other. Therefore, a difference in the outcome variable can be attributable only to the treatment variable.

As we have seen, many interesting questions in medicine cannot be answered by this kind of research design, because the putative causal variable—for instance, smoking—cannot be controlled by an experimenter. For decades, we have been concerned about the effect of smoking on cancer or heart disease, but this cannot be studied experimentally in humans because researchers cannot randomly assign some research participants to smoke and others not to smoke. Therefore, as we have seen, the only approach to studying the health consequences of smoking is to assemble groups that *already differ* in regard to the key variable—in this case, smoking. Thus, researchers assemble groups of smoking and nonsmoking participants and then measure cancer or heart disease to determine if there are systematic differences related to smoking status.

For precisely these reasons, the study of the association between religious attendance and mortality must rely on observational studies. Researchers can no more assign participants to attend religious services frequently or infrequently or not at all than they can make some people smokers and others nonsmokers. When variables cannot be controlled by researchers, as in the case of smoking or attendance at services, all that the researchers can do is to *select* participants who vary in the variable of interest and *observe* what happens to them.

In Chapter 6, we discussed the problems associated with Comstock's study of church attendance and mortality. Remember that Comstock thought he had demonstrated a connection between the two, but it was later discovered to be the product of the failure to control for functional impairment: people who already were sick couldn't get to church and were more likely to die. In observational studies like this one, the fact that subjects self-select makes it very difficult to identify causal contributions. Participants in studies of religious attendance and health are *chosen* on the basis of preexisting characteristics that they themselves select rather than being assigned to different levels of the variable in question, as would be done in an experiment. Groups that are selected on the basis of their differences on a key variable of interest also may differ on variables that are associated with the outcome variable. For instance, people who take a college-preparation course may perform better on an exam than those who don't take the course. This seems to suggest that taking the course is responsible for the differences in the scores. But people *choose* to take the course or not to take it, and these people may differ in significant ways that may explain the differences in their exam scores. Those who choose to take the course may simply be more dedicated than those who don't take it. They may be less fearful of academic activities than those who don't take the course. Either of these two other characteristics—being more dedicated or less intimidated—may account for the differences in scores on the exam. The differences may have nothing whatever to do with the course itself.

These other variables may *confound* the association between the putative causal variable and the outcome variable. This is clearly true of studies of religious attendance. Differences in attendance may be accompanied by a great many other differences that are equally plausibly related to the outcome variable under investigation. For instance, people who are more depressed may be less likely to attend church. People who live alone may be less likely to attend. And, of course, people who are sick may be less likely to attend. All of these other factors may account for the relationship between church attendance and mortality. It may have nothing to do with going to church.

This is the classical problem of self-selection in observational research: people who differ on a key variable in question because they *choose* to behave in a certain way—they *choose* to attend regularly or they *choose* to attend infrequently—are very likely to differ not only in this way but in many other ways, too. Because the groups defined by differences in the key variable also differ in other important respects, we can never be sure that outcome variable differences are attributable to the variable we believe is important and not to another variable.

Epidemiologists have analytical strategies to address this concern. These strategies invariably require the researchers to specify the other variables they believe might function as confounders, i.e., might also be linked to the putative causal variable and also affect the outcome variable, and then attempt to *statistically control* for these differences in the confounding variables. Essentially, this strategy calls for the researchers to determine that the two groups—those who attend frequently and those who don't, or smokers and nonsmokers—differ substantially only in the putative causal variable and not in these other, confounding variables. To use the examples above, researchers would attempt to determine that even after considering the impact on mortality of factors like depression, living alone, and sickness, we *still* find that church attendance is associated with reduced mortality. This technique is applied all the time in epidemiological studies.

The problem with the technique is simple: We have no idea if the variables we specify as potential confounders are the only ones that could influence the outcome variable. For example, contemporary studies of religious attendance and mortality control for age, race, education, income, functional status, social characteristics, and health behavior. When they report that even after controlling for these potential confounders, the attendance-mortality association is still significant, they assume that association is proven. But it is proven only insofar as the researchers have selected *all* of the potential confounding variables and controlled for them statistically. What if, for example, they forgot depression? After all, depression is a clear risk factor for mortality, and depression may be associated with religious attendance. If depression is omitted from the analysis, then the analytic findings are open to question. The problem with observational studies like these is that we can never be certain we have identified all the potential confounding variables and included them in the statistical analyses.

A fascinating example of a serious confound that appears to characterize all studies of attendance at religious services and health outcomes was revealed recently by a paper published in the field of economics. In this paper, researcher Jonathan Gruber, an economist at MIT, constructed an index of religious "density." This index refers to the degree to which communities differ in the representation of different religious denominations. A community with a high degree of religious density is one in which there is relatively little religious diversity.

Using data from the U.S. Census Bureau and the General Social Survey, Gruber showed that high religious density in the context of ethnic diversity was associated with higher degrees of religious attendance. That is, in communities like Boston, in which there is a predominant religion—Catholicism—but substantial ethnic diversity—lots of Italian Catholics, lots of Irish Catholics—religious attendance is higher than in communities with low religious density, e.g., New Haven, which has many Catholics, Protestants, and Jews. Not only does density predict attendance, but, importantly, it also predicts some of the societal benefits that some claim are due to religion, such as economic success, low welfare rates, and greater marital stability. These data suggest that religious density produces both higher attendance rates and these societal benefits. Dr. Gruber's argument is perfectly consistent with the position reviewed earlier: that a third factor accounts for both religious attendance and health.

If Dr. Gruber is right, we can draw the following conclusion: The relationship between attendance and positive health outcomes is *epiphenomenal,* i.e., it occurs because attendance and health are both the product of religious density. There is, according to this analysis, no causal connection between attendance and health. They appear to be linked only because both are the product of this third factor.

At the moment, we don't know precisely what this third factor might be. But in studies that rely on self-selection to produce groups of subjects who attend religious services with different frequencies, we can never be entirely certain that there isn't some other factor we haven't considered that in fact is responsible for the association between attendance and mortality.

## The Methodological Problem of Self-Presentation Bias

Most of the research studies showing relationships between religious attendance and mortality rely on interview methods. This was the case for all of the papers Powell and her colleagues reviewed. Data collection involved interviewers asking questions of participants, either in person or over the telephone. Interviews are effective ways of gathering information about people, but it is important to recognize that they are *social* interactions. We know that social interactions are influenced by a number of important factors. One such factor is the concern people have about how the interviewer will evaluate them. As a result, they shade their answers in ways that they believe will improve the impression they make with the interviewer.

Among researchers, this is called the *self-presentation* bias. It represents the tendency of respondents in an interview situation to convey information about themselves in the best possible light and as related to a traditionally accepted social norm. This sort of bias can influence responses to surveys. It can easily influence how one understands the survey question, the recall of correct information, and how one responds to the question.

In Gallup surveys and the General Social Survey that ask about religious attendance, these questions are posed like this:

- "How often to you attend religious services?"
- "Did you, yourself, happen to attend church or synagogue in the last seven days, or not?"
- "How often do you attend church or synagogue? At least once a week, almost every week, about once a month, seldom, or never?"

Questions like "How often do you attend religious services?" can be understood by people being interviewed in a variety of ways. Though the question asked is "How often do you attend religious services?" the interviewee may hear "Are you a good Christian?" People who think they ought to go to church on a regular basis because of what others may think or because of the way they perceive their religion may be more likely to report that they have attended even if they didn't, in order to present themselves in a better light. This is the essence of self-presentation bias. We all want to be perceived in the best light possible. It's only human, but it poses a problem for researchers.

What is the consequence of self-presentation bias in this context? Considerable evidence suggests that it results in overestimation of attendance rates. People simply report that they attend more often than they actually do.

What is the degree of this overestimation? Can it be measured? Quantifying overestimation requires obtaining a true level of attendance and comparing it with the estimates from surveys. Kirk Hadaway and colleagues did precisely this. They conducted a survey of Ashtabula County, Ohio, and estimated that the county's Protestant population was about 66,500. The survey also revealed that 35.8 percent of the Protestant population reported attendance at religious services during the previous week. These researchers then painstakingly located every church in the county and obtained average attendance information from them using a variety of sources, including telephone interviews, church visits, membership totals, and denominational yearbooks. Based on this information, they calculated that the real attendance rate was only 19.6 percent.

Collecting information in a different way, they concluded that the attendance rate of Catholics was actually about 25 percent instead of the 51 percent derived from a survey. Other researchers of attendance at Catholic services came to the same conclusion. That is, estimates of attendance using methods not subject to self-presentation biases were just slightly more than half of the rate derived from the survey.

Data collected in a completely different way also demonstrate that survey reports of attendance at religious services are overestimated. Rather than raise the risk of self-presentation bias, sociologists Stanley Presser of the University of Maryland and Linda Stinson of the U.S. Bureau of Labor Statistics collected information without ever mentioning attendance at religious services, or any other event, for that matter. That is, they employed a method called *time use estimation*. Using this technique, research participants were not asked about whether or not they engaged in any particular events. Rather, they were asked questions like the following: "I would like to ask you about the things you did yesterday—from midnight Saturday to midnight last night. Let's start with midnight Saturday. What were you doing? What time did you finish? Where were you? What did you do next?" Presser and Stinson compared reports of attendance at religious services derived from data collected in this way on a nationally representative survey in 1993–94 to estimates on attendance from an equally representative national survey conducted over the same time period but measuring attendance at services in the conventional way. Comparing the rates of attendance from the two, they concluded that weekly attendance reports from surveys that used interview methods were overestimated by about 33 percent.

According to Hadaway et al., overestimation of attendance reflects a combination "of a respondent's desire to report *truthfully* his or her identity as a religious, church-going person and the perception that the attendance question is really about this identity rather than about *actual attendance*." Of course, these factors should apply not just to estimates of attendance at religious services but to any socially desirable behavior. This appears to be the case. Estimates of voting behavior and donations to charities, other socially desirable activities, also are overestimated in surveys, presumably because respondents want to look good in the eyes of their interviewers.

Importantly, as self-presentation biases, they are operative in interpersonal situations, i.e., during interviews conducted in person or by telephone. But they may operate less when questions are asked in written format. And they are unlikely to operate when data are collected in ways that do not provoke this bias, i.e., by not asking about events for which social normative pressure exists. Indeed, when questions about attendance were asked only in written format, there was no overestimation.

Tellingly, all of the studies in Powell's review that showed a relationship between religious attendance and mortality used interview methods, either in person or by telephone. We should expect that in all of these studies, reports of attendance were overestimated, and probably by the margins seen in the studies discussed above.

To be honest, we don't know what the impact of such overestimation might be on the attendance-mortality link. It could increase the strength of the relationship, reduce or eliminate it, or leave it unchanged. But demonstrations of overestimation of attendance ought to make us cautious about drawing conclusions from studies showing relationships between religious attendance and health outcomes.

## What Does Attendance at Religious Services Mean?

The reason there are so many studies of attendance at religious services is because it is easy to measure and because it is thought to *represent an underlying degree of religiosity*. Researchers in this area regard attendance as an index of religious involvement that is easy to measure. For example, McCullough et al. entitled their paper that reviewed studies of attendance and mortality "Religious Involvement and Mortality" because they view attendance as an *index* of religious involvement.

But it is immediately apparent that people attend religious services for a great many reasons. Garrison Keillor is reported to have remarked that "anyone who believes that sitting in church will make you a Christian must also believe that sitting in a garage makes you a car." People may attend religious services because of social pressure from family, friends, and neighbors. They may do so out of habit. They may attend because it is a way to meet new people socially. They may attend because it provides valuable business connections. And, of course, they may attend because of religious conviction. There undoubtedly are other reasons, too.

Attending religious services is a *behavior* and may reflect many different underlying motivations. It is easy to measure, but its meaning is unclear.

In this sense, researchers who select attendance at religious services because it is an easy-to-measure predictor variable are like the proverbial drunk who looks for his lost wallet under the streetlight, not because he thinks he lost it there but because that's where the light is better. Attendance is seen as relatively easy to measure accurately, so researchers use it as an index of religiosity. But because it may reflect so many different motivations, it becomes difficult to know how to interpret relationships between attendance and health.

This questionable relationship between the measurable index, attendance at religious services, and the underlying factor it presumably reflects, religious devotion or faith, represents a central issue in science: *construct validity.* In this case, the underlying construct is religious devotion. But it's underlying, i.e., it's not something like hair color or weight or blood pressure that we can measure directly. The best we can do is to consider easily measurable *indices* that presumably reflect the underlying construct. But the index we measure is not the same as the underlying construct. As we saw above, attending religious services can mean many things, only one of which is religious devotion.

Of course, this doesn't mean that attendance *never* reflects devotion. That's obviously not the case. But it does mean that attendance and devotion are not equivalent. Attendance is an imperfect index of devotion.

This kind of measurement imperfection is common in the social sciences, and once again we can turn to Stephen Jay Gould for a wonderful example. In his classic book *The Mismeasure of Man,* Gould addressed the difference between IQ and intelligence. *Intelligence* is an underlying construct. *IQ* is established by the result of a person's performance on an IQ test. It is a score. While we may believe that IQ tells us something about intelligence, we recognize that IQ *is not the same as* intelligence. It is an index that only imperfectly reflects the underlying construct. In Chapter 6, we saw that in the early twentieth century in the U.S., the measurement of IQ was heavily influenced by the degree of familiarity with American culture. Immigrant groups less familiar with U.S. culture performed more poorly on IQ tests. Their relatively poor performance reflected the fact that IQ is only partially related to intelligence. Because we can't directly access intelligence to measure it, we must rely on indirect and imperfect indices.

Like intelligence, religious devotion, religious involvement, and religiosity are constructs that we may recognize as important but that are not directly accessible. Because of this, we cannot measure them directly. We can only infer their dimensions indirectly using indices that we believe reflect them. But just as IQ only imperfectly reflects intelligence, so attendance at religious services only imperfectly reflects religiosity or religious devotion.

## Do Observational Studies Linking Attendance and Mortality Have Anything to Say About Medical Treatment?

Epidemiological studies in medicine aim to identify factors that cause disease so that they can inform medical practice and public health.

The most celebrated epidemiological studies having an impact on the popular consciousness in the past several decades are those that looked at the effects of smoking. Epidemiological associations between smoking and cancer and heart disease were so solid that medical practice was altered. Physicians now routinely ask their patients about smoking and recommend to their patients who still smoke that they quit. Epidemiological associations between low-fat diets high in fruits and vegetables, and reduced rates of cardiovascular disease have led to dietary recommendations that are routinely offered by physicians. The point of these studies and others like them is to develop evidence about risks to health that can form the basis of physician recommendations to patients in the service of improving their health.

Even if none of the problems with the relationship between religious service attendance and mortality existed, physicians would still not be justified in recommending that their patients attend religious services or become more religious in general, for several reasons. First, attendance may reflect a great many different motives, and we have no idea which of them might be associated with the mortality effect. A similar problem does not exist in recommendations to consume a low-fat diet or to stop smoking, largely because there is no ambiguity about the underlying meaning about fruit and vegetable consumption or smoking. Moreover, because we can also investigate the smoking-disease connection on cells and tissues in the laboratory and in animal studies, the physiological connections between smoking and disease are reasonably well understood. And correspondingly, even if there are multiple reasons why someone would eat a low-fat diet (to be healthy, to lose weight, likes the taste), the role that these different motivations play in the physiology is largely irrelevant to the mechanism of the effect. Not so with religious attendance.

For this reason, recommending religious attendance and recommending a low-fat diet to patients are quite different. We know from the considerable research on adherence to medical recommendations that patients vary considerably in the degree to which they follow the recommendations of physicians. We have no idea whether patients would follow a physician's recommendation to attend religious services more frequently. The same, of course, is true of all other physician recommendations, but there is a critical difference between a recommendation to attend services and a recommendation to eat a low-fat diet. This difference derives from our understanding of the mechanism by which a low-fat diet influences the underlying pathophysiology of, for example, diabetes or heart disease, and our corresponding lack of understanding of what religious attendance means and therefore how it might have a physiological impact.

And because we have no idea what attending services means to patients, we have no idea whether attending because your physician recommends it would have the same effect as attending because you have chosen it for yourself.

Of course, there is another major difference between recommending a low-fat diet and recommending attendance at religious services. In the U.S., we have a tradition of freedom of religious expression. Physician recommendations to engage in religious activity of any sort have the potential to be manipulative or even coercive and so threaten this religious freedom. The U.S. Constitution and the Bill of Rights do not protect our right to select a diet of our choice.

## WHAT CAN WE SAY, THEN, ABOUT THE CONNECTIONS BETWEEN RELIGIOUS ATTENDANCE AND MORTALITY, IF ANYTHING?

As we have seen, the claims about the number of studies relevant to the health benefits of active religious involvement are exaggerated. In fact, although the literature on religion and health may be large, a great many of these studies are about matters not relevant to health benefits of religious involvement. And among those that truly are relevant, a great many fail to meet the standards of research methodology that would give us confidence in their findings. Even accepting the view of Powell and colleagues that the evidence linking attendance at religious services to reduced mortality is persuasive, we have seen that attending services may mean many different things and, moreover, that surveys that collect information by interviews tend to substantially overestimate attendance, largely due to self-presentation bias. An imprecise estimate of the variable most strongly linked to a health outcome does not give us much confidence in these findings. Overall, the evidence linking religious involvement and health outcomes remains weak and inconclusive. It is still a work in progress and by no means justifies any changes in clinical medicine.

# 9

## WHY LONG-DISTANCE HEALING
## DOESN'T HAVE A PRAYER

**Most of the interest in religion and health has cen-**tered on the question of whether the religious involvement of individuals benefits their own health. Everyone wants to know if people who attend religious services or read the Bible regularly are more likely to be healthy than those who do so infrequently or not at all. In this chapter we will consider a much more controversial—even revolutionary—proposal: that our health can be affected by the thoughts or intentions of others, which has been referred to as *distant healing* or *distant intentionality,* or by their prayers, which has been referred to as *intercessory prayer.* Of course, we'll have a critical look at the studies that purport to prove that these phenomena exist. This is no small matter because if such studies do indeed confirm their existence, it would provide powerful ammunition to those who say that religious activities should have a greater role in the practice of medicine. Beyond that, it would pose a challenge to our understanding of consciousness and the physical universe.

Intercessory prayer (IP) has commanded most of the attention in recent years. In these studies, intercessors pray for a randomly selected sample of patients, usually at a considerable distance from the intercessors, while a control group of patients receives no such prayer. Both groups are then assessed according to some specific health outcomes. In several widely publicized studies, researchers reported that the prayers of the intercessors did indeed result in better health outcomes for the prayer subjects compared to the control groups. Other studies have shown no effect of prayer, but some of the authors appear undaunted in their advocacy. The entirely negative results of the largest study of IP yet undertaken have just been released.

Studies of IP provide one great advantage over the ones we reviewed in previous chapters. In those, researchers were unable to control the religious involvement that would presumably influence health outcomes in the participants. Because it would be impossible to take a group of people and randomly make one half of them religious and the other half not religious, the only way of conducting those studies was to *select* groups of subjects who *already differed* in their degree of religious involvement. As we saw, this raises numerous methodological problems, especially the problem of self-selection: people who are dissimilar in their religious practices may also differ from each other in many other ways, and it may be these other characteristics rather than a person's religious practices that account for any differences in health.

Those who study IP don't have this problem. They can conduct a true experiment in which research subjects are assigned to a treatment condition on a random basis. By the flip of a coin or a computer-generated schedule of numbers, they can assign subjects randomly either to receive standard medical care as well as the prayers of a group of distant intercessors, or to receive standard medical care alone.

This means—assuming that there is a large enough sample—that there is a reasonable degree of certainty that all the differences between the two groups of subjects have been eliminated except for the one independent variable: prayer. So if a well-conducted experiment on IP turns out to yield a significant health advantage to the prayer group over the control group, the difference can safely be attributed to prayer. Unfortunately, this methodological advantage has been squandered, outweighed by other serious shortcomings. Let's look at several of the most prominent examples.

## THE FAMOUS STUDY OF DR. RANDOLPH BYRD

The best-known study of the impact of distant IP was conducted in the mid-1980s by Randolph Byrd, a San Francisco cardiologist. Published in 1988 in the *Southern Medical Journal,* the paper reports that 393 patients in the coronary care unit (CCU) of a San Francisco hospital were assigned randomly to receive either standard medical care or this same standard care plus daily IP from three to seven born-again Christians. Byrd recorded differences between the two groups on twenty-nine outcome variables that characterized the course of recovery in the CCU. For example, he contrasted the prayer and control group on the use of antianginal agents (drugs to control chest pain and shortness of breath), antiarrhythmic medications (drugs that treat irregular heart rhythms), the need for arterial pressure monitoring (putting a catheter in an artery), the need for diuretics, whether they developed pneumonia, and whether they required a pacemaker. He reported that on six of these twenty-nine variables—the development of congestive heart failure, the use of a diuretic, cardiopulmonary arrest (your heart stops and you stop breathing), pneumonia, the need for antibiotics, and requiring mechanical assistance for breathing—the prayer group had a superior outcome.

At first glance it seems as if the study did demonstrate that prayer worked, but a closer examination shows something else. First there is the problem of multiple comparisons, something we've already discussed in Chapter 6. Each time you conduct a statistical test, you increase the likelihood that a chance finding will be misinterpreted as real. By conducting twenty-nine different statistical tests (one for each of the twenty-nine variables measured), Byrd virtually assured that he would mistake chance findings for real effects of prayer. So his finding that the prayer group was less likely to develop pneumonia than the control group is more likely due to chance than to prayer. In fact, if Byrd had adjusted his criterion of statistical significance to control for the number of tests he conducted, the critical probability to rule out chance would have been 0.0017 (nearly 1 in 500), not 0.05 (1 in 20) as he claimed. This means all of Byrd's findings were most likely the result of chance alone. They had nothing to do with prayer.

To make matters worse, the six "significant" outcomes were not independent of each other. Two of the categories were newly diagnosed cases of heart failure and newly prescribed diuretics. There were fewer cases of each in the prayer group. But diuretics are routinely prescribed for heart failure, so these two variables really measure the same thing. Similarly, the prayer group had fewer newly diagnosed cases of pneumonia and fewer newly prescribed antibiotics, but these aren't independent variables either, because antibiotics are prescribed for pneumonia.

So, aside from the problem of multiple comparisons, there really were only four and not six variables on which the two groups differed significantly: heart failure, cardiopulmonary arrest, pneumonia, and mechanical assistance for breathing. In addition, there was no difference between the two groups for some other important variables: days in the CCU, length of stay in the hospital, and number of discharge medications.

In this study, therefore, of the great many comparisons made between the prayer and the standard-care groups, only a very few appeared to reflect a statistically significant difference, and—if accepted research methodology standards had been followed—even those few could not be considered significant.

# THE HARRIS STUDY

Less well known but methodologically superior to Byrd's study, the investigation by Dr. William Harris and colleagues published in 1999 was a relatively well-conducted IP investigation. It had all the characteristics—randomized, controlled, double-blind, prospective—of a good randomized controlled trial. And, unlike the Byrd study, this paper was published in a first-rate journal, the respected *Archives of Internal Medicine*.

It reported the effects of IP on two criteria—adverse events and length of hospital stay—in 990 patients admitted to the CCU in a Kansas City hospital. The patients were assigned on a completely random basis to receive standard care or remote IP in addition to standard care.

The delivery of the prayer was tightly controlled by the experimenters: Teams of Christian intercessors received the first names of patients in the prayer group and were instructed to pray for these patients to have a speedy recovery; only those in the treatment group received these prayers. The intercessors were to pray on a daily basis for four weeks. Both the patients and those who evaluated their medical conditions were "blinded," kept unaware of who was being prayed for. The study was also prospective, meaning that the patients were followed after the intervention to determine if the group receiving the prayer had better outcomes in the CCU. These elements of the experimental design are first-rate.

The problems with the study emerge from the way the researchers considered the outcome variables. Harris and colleagues constructed a new way of measuring how well the patients did in the CCU. They collected information on the various medical events that might occur. Patients might need antibiotics, arterial monitoring, drugs to control angina. They could require more complex interventions, including invasive procedures to identify the source of a cardiac arrhythmia. They could die. In all, the investigators identified thirty-five events, and for each assigned a value or weight that corresponded to what *they perceived* as the seriousness of each event. Thus, the need for a procedure to identify the source of an arrhythmia was given three points, while the need for antibiotics was assigned a single point. Death rated six points. To evaluate their new scale, they asked ten colleagues in cardiology to determine if they agreed on the weighting of the thirty-five events and reported that these colleagues agreed 96 percent of the time.

Having constructed this new scale, the researchers then compared the prayer and control groups in two ways: using a weighted and unweighted scale. In the former, they calculated the average number of points for each patient in the two groups and compared them. Using this approach, they found that the prayer group had a significantly better course of recovery in the CCU, that is, a lower total of points for adverse events than the control group.

Using the latter approach, the researchers simply counted the number of adverse events per patient in the two groups and then compared them. That is, using an unweighted index, one event counted as much as the next: the need for antibiotics counted as much as the need for an invasive arrhythmia procedure or even death. On this index, too, the prayer group had a significant advantage.

On other indices, including a measure based on the Byrd study, and length of stay in the CCU and in the hospital, the two groups did not differ. Based on these findings, Harris and colleagues boldly stated, "This result suggests that prayer may be an effective adjunct to standard medical care."

On the surface, these findings, like those of Byrd, are striking because they suggest that the researchers had been able to document an effect of IP. As might be expected, a considerable controversy arose surrounding this publication. In fact, as an editor of the *Archives of Internal Medicine* reported to me at the time, the article stimulated more letters to the editor than any other paper in the history of the journal.

My colleague Emilia Bagiella and I wrote one of those letters which, along with many others, was published in 2000. Our letter was entitled "Data Without a Prayer." We pointed out, first of all, that despite the fact that the intercessors prayed only for a speedy recovery, the prayer group did not recover faster than the control group.

We also identified another subtle but important problem: the scale that was constructed to measure clinical course in the CCU. Harris and his coauthors wrote that their scale was acceptable because their cardiology colleagues agreed with the weights or values assigned to the various events that could occur in the CCU. In the language of research methodology, these researchers confused *inter-rater reliability* with *construct validity*. Inter-rater reliability refers to the degree to which different people will agree on the measurement of something. For instance, IQ tests are said to have high inter-rater reliability because different people who administer them to the same people generally report the same results. Construct validity, on the other hand, addresses the degree to which the measurement scale accurately reflects what it purports to measure. To take the example of IQ again, if we wanted to determine the construct validity of an IQ test, we would have to answer the question of whether or not the test accurately measures that intellectual capacity. Of course, that question is fraught with controversy, but I think you can see what I mean. In the case of the Harris study, for the scale to have construct validity it would have to accurately reflect the degree of problems in recovering in the CCU. This is very different from determining whether people agree on a measurement strategy.

As we pointed out in our letter, the unweighted scale used by Harris and colleagues was completely meaningless, as their own example illustrated: a patient who dies right away in the CCU has a better unweighted score (one event) than a patient who survives but requires antibiotics, arterial monitoring, and anti-anginal agents (three events). Clearly dying is not one of the desired outcomes in the CCU, while survival—even after many different treatments—is.

The difference between the two groups using the weighted scale is significant only if it has construct validity. In this experiment, the need for an invasive arrhythmia procedure was assigned three points. But is that outcome really three times as bad as the need for antibiotics, which was assigned one point? How do we know that it is three times as bad? Why isn't it four times as bad? Or only twice as bad? In fact, we don't know. Because of this, the scale used in this study does not have established validity. We can't rely on it to assess accurately what it purports to measure. High inter-rater reliability is not a substitute for construct validity. Harris and colleagues suggest that the high inter-rater agreement (96 percent) on the scores for eleven randomly selected cases addresses this matter, but it does not. As we pointed out in our letter, raters might also agree substantially on hair color, but that does not make it a meaningful clinical index.

Thus, although better controlled and executed than the Byrd study, the Harris study also suffers from serious methodological problems that cast doubt on its findings. Like the Byrd study, it too fails to prove an effect of IP.

## THE MANTRA STUDY

In Chapter 7, we briefly discussed the MANTRA pilot study. Let's revisit it now, then go on to a more thorough examination of the recently published full study, MANTRA II.

In the pilot study, 150 patients with acute coronary syndromes who were undergoing angioplasty were assigned at random to receive one of five conditions:

1. Imagery
2. Touch therapy
3. Stress relaxation
4. Distant intercessory prayer
5. Standard care

Authors Dr. Mitchell Krucoff and colleagues collected many outcome variables including myocardial ischemia, heart rate variability, adverse events after the procedure, and mortality. Myocardial ischemia refers to a lack of blood flow to the heart, a potentially serious medical problem. Circulating blood is the source of oxygen to all the tissues of the body, and if the blood supply is interrupted or reduced for some reason, the tissues becomes starved for oxygen. In the case of the heart muscle, this condition may be accompanied by chest pain or shortness of breath.

Heart rate variability is a measure of how the nervous system controls the heart. It's good to have a lot of heart rate variability. The adverse events following the angioplasty included death, heart failure, myocardial infarction (a heart attack), or the need to repeat the angioplasty or undergo bypass surgery.

The results of the pilot study were entirely negative. There were no statistically significant differences between the groups in myocardial ischemia, heart rate variability, or adverse events. However, because this was a *pilot* study, it is appropriate to look at differences between the groups that fail to reach statistical significance so that you can plan a larger study that can be more definitive. Krucoff and colleagues reported that when all the alternative treatment groups were combined, they had a 25 to 30 percent lower rate of adverse events compared with the standard-care group. Again, this difference wasn't statistically significant, but the authors reasoned that it might be worth conducting a larger study to examine it.

The authors also compared the alternative treatments among themselves and reported that while patients were still hospitalized after the procedure, the prayer group had the lowest rate of adverse events. Again comparing the alternative treatments to each other, the prayer condition was associated with fewer deaths while in the hospital and during the six-month follow-up. But again, none of these differences was significant. The authors also reported that all of the deaths in the study came in the alternative treatment groups. No one in the standard-care condition died. This finding, too, did not achieve statistical significance, but it came closer to significance than any other. In this respect, the alternative treatments were *more* dangerous than standard care.

On the basis of these pilot study findings, Krucoff and co-investigators began MANTRA II, designed to be the *definitive* study. It was to be substantially larger than the pilot study and therefore could adequately test the hypotheses. In MANTRA II, 748 patients undergoing angioplasty or cardiac catheterization at nine sites in the U.S. were randomized to one of four conditions:

1. Standard care
2. Distant intercessory prayer
3. A combination of music, guided imagery, and touch (MIT)
4. Prayer plus MIT

End points included major adverse cardiovascular events, readmission to the hospital, or death within the first six months of follow-up. The authors were also interested in these same outcomes in the next six months. By major adverse cardiovascular events, they meant a new heart attack, new heart failure, repeat angioplasty, or coronary artery bypass surgery.

The findings from MANTRA II were published in the *Lancet,* one of the most prestigious journals in medicine. It was accompanied by an editorial praising the trial. Analysis of the data revealed no differences whatsoever between the groups on any of these primary or secondary end points. Krucoff and colleagues also measured the distress that patients reported before the medical procedure and found that this distress was lower in the MIT group. Mortality at six months also was lower for the MIT group.

In other words, there was no effect at all of distant prayer on any of the outcome variables measured in MANTRA II. In the discussion section of the paper, the authors could have concluded that because they had conducted a definitive study, it was now time to abandon efforts to demonstrate scientifically the effect of distant prayer.

They didn't. Virtually the entire discussion section of the paper was devoted to the topic of distant prayer. After the obligatory reiteration of the fact that prayer for the sick is practiced throughout the world, the authors then went on to inform the readers that the mechanisms through which distant prayer might work are unknown, blithely ignoring the fact that they had just demonstrated that *it didn't work*. They continued, exploring data from other studies of intercessory prayer, and in an attempt to salvage their hypothesis, they questioned whether the outcome would have been different if elements of the intercessory interventions had differed. Would it have made a difference if the prayers had come from individuals rather than congregations? Would the prayers of different religions have had different effects? Was the number of individuals praying important? Were the timing and duration of the prayers important?

Before the study had completed data collection, Dr. Krucoff declared that MANTRA II would be the *definitive* study of distant intercessory prayer. According to a news release from Duke University, the results of the MANTRA pilot study were promising enough to warrant a definitive investigation. Apparently, once Krucoff saw that the findings were entirely negative, he thought better of this statement and wrote about using secondary data analysis from MANTRA II as a guide for future trials of distant prayer. That is, now MANTRA II also would be regarded as a pilot study on which another "definitive" study would be based.

Drs. Krucoff and colleagues deserve credit for conducting a truly well-controlled and well-designed test of the impact of distant prayer on medical outcomes. MANTRA II is, as he originally commented, a definitive study. It definitively demonstrates that there is no effect of distant prayer.

One other element of MANTRA II deserves mention. We saw above that the researchers questioned whether the prayers of different religious traditions might have different effects. In an editorial accompanying the report of MANTRA II, *The Lancet* asked precisely the same question, suggesting that we should conduct such a test. It is hard to imagine a more troubling recommendation. Even if there were a plausible mechanism to account for possible effects of distant prayer, do we really want to test denominational differences in its efficacy? Theological critics of this kind of research have for years objected to putting God to the test. In a world riven with fundamentalist religious strife, attempting to show the superiority of one form of prayer over another is not only offensive but dangerous.

## OTHER STUDIES, OTHER PROBLEMS

There are other papers claiming to show effects of IP. Like those already examined, they are characterized by significant methodological problems that raise questions about their conclusions. Of course there are also papers that report the opposite finding, that IP has no effect. As I edit this section of the book, the negative results of the biggest IP study yet, the Study of the Therapeutic Effects of Intercessory Prayer (STEP study), directed by Herbert Benson at Harvard, have just been published. In this study, as in MANTRA II, distant prayer had no effect.

This $2.4 million study, funded by the John Templeton Foundation, was a multicenter trial of 1,802 patients recovering from coronary artery bypass graft surgery in six U.S. hospitals and randomized to one of three groups: one that was informed it might or might not receive prayer from distant intercessors and did in fact receive prayer; a second that was informed it might or might not receive prayer and did not receive prayer; and a third that was informed it would receive prayer and did receive it as promised. The third group was added to control for the possibility that it might be the *expectation* that one would receive prayer rather than the prayer itself that could have an impact on outcomes. A fourth possible group that would have expected to receive prayer but then did not receive prayer was properly deemed ethically unacceptable by the researchers.

Intercessors, who came from three mainstream religious groups, began their prayers for patients assigned to receive them on the night before surgery and continued them for two weeks. Data were collected from January 1998 to November 2000. Those of us who follow this research wondered why it took six years after the completion of data collection to report the findings. We also should wonder why over $2 million was spent studying the effects of prayer rather than trying to improve the delivery of treatments that have been proven effective.

Beyond these specific problems, there is another general problem that fatally compromises IP studies. Although they permit random assignment of subjects to the prayer and control conditions, this advantage is lost because of the inability of the experimenters to control exposure of subjects to other sources of prayer. Ideally, only the treatment group would receive prayers for their health, while the control subjects would receive none at all, just as in a study of a new medication, the treatment group receives a specified amount of the drug, and the control group receives only a placebo or no treatment at all. But in IP studies, the treatment and control groups differ only in the prayers said on their behalf *by the designated intercessors,* not in prayers from family and friends, from fellow members of their religious congregations, and from religious orders who pray for all the sick all over the world. Indeed, the volume of "prayer noise," as some of the IP researchers describe the prayer of people other than the designated intercessors, is likely to be considerably greater than that of the intercessors.

Consider the case of the Harris study. The authors reported that each subject received a daily prayer from five intercessors for twenty-eight days. However, the outcome measures concerned clinical course in the coronary care unit, and the average length of stay in the CCU was only 1.1 days. Thus, exposure to distant intercessory prayer could not have exceeded, on average, six prayers before the outcome variables were measured. It is not difficult to imagine how the supplementary prayer from friends, relatives, and members of the patients' religious congregations would exceed this amount. In such a study, should we ask these people not to pray for the patient? If not, how could we interpret a hypothetical outcome in which an IP group improves to a greater degree than the control group? Do the prayers of the intercessors somehow carry more weight than those of the much larger group of others who pray? Why should this be so?

This problem is a specific instance of a more general failure of IP studies. We have no idea how to quantify or specify the dimensions of the central independent variable: prayer. Without this information we are unable to determine the degree of exposure to prayer, and therefore we can draw no firm conclusions about outcomes. Continuing the analogy with research on the effect of medication, it is as if the effectiveness of a drug was also being studied without regard for either its purity, the quantity being consumed, or the degree to which subjects in the control group also were taking the drug.

Jeffrey Dusek and colleagues from the STEP study acknowledge this limitation but nonetheless proceeded with their research. They write that their study examines the impact of "additional intercessory prayer." By describing it as "additional," they have recognized the problem of others praying for their research subjects.

This recognition itself, however, raises other significant issues, by implying that prayer has certain properties. At the very least, the idea of "additional" prayer suggests that prayer has quantity; that there can be more or less of it; and that, presumably, its effect is a function of quantity, so that greater amounts of prayer are more effective than smaller amounts. Moreover, the "volume" of prayer by the limited number of intercessors is certain to be dwarfed by the considerably greater "prayer noise," but Dusek and colleagues imply that the small increment provided by the intercessors nevertheless can have significant clinical impact. At the very least, these implications should be examined.

IP studies also raise significant conceptual problems. Assuming there were effects, what mechanism could be responsible for them? That is, *how* could the prayers of one group of people affect the physical health of another group of people at a great distance? Although many possible mechanisms have been proposed by researchers, two have received the most attention: divine intervention and distant effects (the thoughts and intentions of people producing effects at a great distance).

Several groups of scholars have written critically about attributing the effect of IP studies to divine intervention, arguing that it is unlikely that a god would disadvantage patients randomly assigned to a control group simply because an experimenter wanted to prove a point. Why, this criticism goes, would God intervene to cause some randomly selected patients to have a poorer course of recovery than others simply to support the hypothesis of a scientist? Why would God submit to such a test? Do we really believe in such a capricious deity? As Stephen Black put it, we should hope that this is not the case.

If we reject the notion of divine intervention, then the alternative is that a human mechanism—distant healing—would be involved. That is, the cognitive activities of one or more people influence the physical well-being of a remote group of patients.

## WEAK AND STRONG CLAIMS FOR IP

Supporters of distant healing make both weak and strong claims. The weak version holds that we should accept the findings of IP studies even if we currently have no understanding of the mechanisms that might explain them. Larry Dossey, a prominent proponent of this view, compares IP to the treatment of scurvy by consumption of citrus fruit, which occurred long before we understood that the vitamin C in the fruit was the responsible mechanism. Dr. Mitchell Krucoff, the principal investigator of the MANTRA studies, agrees with this position. He argues that our lack of knowledge underlying causal mechanisms should not impede the examination of interesting research findings. He and Dr. Dossey are right, of course. Many medical treatments have been used effectively before we understood the underlying mechanisms. But there is a critical difference between the medical treatment they refer to and IP. The critical difference is that there was ample evidence from methodologically acceptable studies about the efficacy of these other treatments. We cannot say that about IP.

Needless to say, IP researchers disagree. The IP findings are so strong, they believe, that we not only must accept them while we await the discovery of the operative mechanism but also must incorporate them into the practice of medicine. As Dossey puts it, "We need not wait until all the answers are in before employing prayer adjunctively." Dr. William Harris also recommends prayer as "an effective adjunct to standard medical care."

The absence of underlying theory raises a significant problem for these claims. IP studies typically collect data on a great many outcome variables. The Byrd, Harris, and STEP studies collected twenty-nine, thirty-nine, and thirty-six outcome variables respectively. Because of the lack of an underlying theory, these studies do not specify which of these many outcome variables should be influenced by prayer. Why, in the Byrd study, should the effect be seen in heart failure but not cardiac arrhythmias? Why, despite the fact that both the Byrd and Harris studies examined clinical course in the CCU, were the findings from the two studies different? This again is the problem of the sharpshooter's fallacy: searching through the data until a significant effect is found, then drawing the bull's-eye. And why, as some observers have suggested, do IP studies examine only relatively trivial outcome variables like the need for antibiotics instead of really important ones like survival, as Dr. Joseph Chibnall recommends? The lack of a theory about the operative mechanisms encourages fishing expeditions and raises the problem of multiple comparisons, which we noted earlier.

The strong claim frames the existence of IP and DH as consistent with new trends in the philosophy of consciousness and quantum mechanics. "While it is true that there is no generally accepted theory for the remote actions of consciousness, many mathematicians, physicists, and biological and cognitive scientists are currently offering hypotheses about how these events may happen," Dossey writes about IP. And "there is considerable evidence that neither telepathy nor psychokinesis (the ability to use mental powers to move objects) is nonsense."

This argument raises considerably greater problems related to our understanding of both consciousness and the physical universe. Consciousness is seen not only to have effects on physical processes but to exert them at a distance. If accepted, the distant-healing literature requires that we abandon the way in which we understand ourselves and the universe, something we should not do in the absence of truly compelling evidence. Exceptional claims require exceptional evidence.

It is true indeed that philosophers have long considered the problem of how consciousness, with no physical properties, could arise from the brain, a physical substrate. In this sense, consciousness is *nonlocal,* dependent upon but apparently not residing in the brain. But asserting that consciousness is nonlocal in this way is considerably different from asserting that it can influence physical or biological phenomena, even those close by, let alone those at a great distance. Nothing in currently accepted views of consciousness permits such an assertion.

It is also true that quantum mechanics considers nonlocal effects. Under certain experimental conditions, the spin of two photons deriving from the same excited atom is consistently related, even if the photons exist at a distance from each other. Thus, the effect is nonlocal. But physicists emphasize that the photons are related merely in a *correlational* and not a *causal* way. Neither photon is seen as causing the behavior of the other. So while quantum physics posits the existence of nonlocal effects, they cannot be the basis of health outcomes seen as *causally* linked to antecedent prayer or other distant intentions.

In nature there are only four basic forces, and none is capable of accounting for the IP effects. The first two—strong and weak nuclear forces—have effects only at the subatomic level. The third, gravitational force, acts at a distance but only in proportion to the masses involved. The mass of the brain, indeed of an entire person, is so trivially small that no effect of gravity could account for how the thoughts of a person in Baltimore could influence the health of another person in Detroit. Electromagnetic energy, the fourth basic force, is associated with brain activity and conceivably could account for IP effects, but this too is unlikely: The electrical activity of the brain, measured at the surface of the skull, is tiny (about $10^{-4}$ volts), and the brain's magnetic field is even smaller than that. Neither can be detected at a distance of even a few feet, even by our most sensitive instruments, let alone at hundreds of miles. Proponents of IP must explain how their findings can be reconciled with these facts or, alternatively, why they do not apply.

## REVOLUTIONARY SCIENCE

The research that claims to prove an IP effect represents, for its proponents, nothing short of a scientific revolution. They embellish their published work with allusions to breakthroughs of the past. They compare IP findings to the work of Newton, for example, both in the inability of the contemporary science to embrace it and in the scorn he received from the established scientific community.

Newton, of course, gave us the principles of celestial mechanics which to this day govern our everyday physical world. In accepting his model, science abandoned its previous beliefs. Science progresses by the accumulation of data that force us, however unwillingly, to relinquish one view in favor of another more consistent with the data. When the mass of data inconsistent with a current view is sufficiently great, we are forced to conclude that the prevailing paradigm is wrong, and a new view takes hold. This is how successive views of the universe, from the Ptolemaic to the Copernican to the Newtonian, evolved.

On the other hand, there have been many claims of revolutionary scientific discoveries throughout history, but only a very few where the data justified those claims. Proponents of IP argue that this criticism is precisely what Newton confronted, and his critics turned out to be wrong. Indeed, how are we to distinguish discoveries that truly represent revolutionary science from those that do not?

One could argue that IP research is at an early stage and we should wait years or decades to see if solid data turn up to support IP before we either embrace or reject it. But not all great scientific advances required decades to be accepted. Einstein's special theory of relativity was accepted within only a few years after publication, and the general theory was accepted almost instantly.

Moreover, there is a critical distinction between scientific revolutions of the past and the IP research. Past revolutions transformed our understanding of phenomena through the formulation of a *theory* that allowed for a new, more thorough and elegant explanation of them than was previously possible.

Darwin's work, for example, provided a comprehensive and radical transformation of our understanding of how living creatures evolve. Newtonian celestial mechanics and Einstein's relativity also accounted for previously inexplicable phenomena. Theories permit these kinds of new understanding and, as a result, the prediction of specific, testable, and potentially disconfirming events.

Following the principles of Newton's mechanics, scientists could predict the precise position of the planet Jupiter on any given date and verify the accuracy of their prediction. This kind of verification supported the theory. Nothing in the IP literature comes remotely close to such an achievement. Not only has no comprehensive theory emerged to account for these findings, but on the contrary, the proponents of IP and DH cannot even specify which of the many outcome variables they collect will be influenced by prayer. Perhaps, if the field develops and new hypotheses emerge that are supported through proper testing, a comprehensive theory will emerge. But until that happens, we shouldn't revise our current understanding of consciousness and the universe. Remember Robert Park's admonitions about claims of revolutionary science.

There is a delicious irony in the treatment of evidence and theory by Dr. William Harris, whose IP study we examined above. In the case of IP, Harris is so willing to accept its efficacy, despite the obvious weaknesses of the studies and data, that he recommends including it in clinical medicine. On the other hand, as managing director of the Intelligent Design Network, an organization that questions Darwinian evolution, Harris is willing to disregard the absolutely voluminous amount of evidence supporting the theory of evolution in order to support intelligent design, a position that has no evidentiary support whatsoever.

Consider also the stance of Dr. Randolph Byrd, the author of the first large IP study. In the acknowledgments section of his study, Byrd credits God's participation in his study. Byrd's acknowledgment and Harris's unwillingness to accept mountains of evidence when it contradicts divine intervention and his willingness to ignore extremely poor-quality evidence when it supports such intervention should make us worry about the motivations of the scientists who conduct studies of IP. As we saw above, science and religion are independent approaches to knowledge, and neither is reducible to the other. When scientists abandon evidence in favor of faith, they no longer operate as scientists.

Every major IP study reporting a positive outcome has serious methodological flaws, and because of them, no evidence exists that prayer by one group of people has an effect on the health of another group. This should make us very cautious indeed about attempts to bring prayer into medical practice.

Of course, this conclusion says nothing about whether people should engage in prayer for reasons of religion. As with other religious practices, science has nothing whatsoever to say about the religious benefits of prayer, whether for oneself or for others. But it can and must say that we have no evidence of the health benefits of distant intercessory prayer.

# PART THREE

Religion and the Practice of Medicine

# 10

## ETHICAL PROBLEMS

## HOW CAN IT HURT?

Early in my research career, I was interviewing a young woman in her hospital room while she awaited the results of a gynecologic biopsy to determine if she had cancer. She shared the semiprivate room with another young woman, also awaiting biopsy results. While the family of this other woman was visiting, a physician entered the room to report that the other woman's biopsy was negative; she did not have cancer. She and her family were greatly relieved, and her father, to no one in particular, exclaimed, "We're good people. We deserve this."

Of course, this was a perfectly natural expression of relief on the part of the patient's father. His daughter was healthy, and he attributed that good news to some kind of cosmic justice from a higher power. But what about the young woman I was interviewing, whose biopsy came back positive? How should she interpret her results? Should she conclude that she had cancer because she was a bad person, because she hadn't been sufficiently faithful? How would you like to be in that young woman's position?

Consider another situation. There is a great deal of evidence that marital status is associated with health. The data generally suggest that both men and women live longer if they are married than if they are not. So if you were an unmarried woman, how would you feel if your physician informed you of this risk—that because you were single, your life expectancy was shortened—and then recommended that you consider finding a husband because of the life-extending effects of marriage? Would you be happy if your doctor recommended that you marry because the evidence suggests that you'll live longer? Do you think doctors should give this kind of advice to patients?

And here's a third situation to consider. Not only have recent research studies examined the association between religious practices and health, but some of these studies have even gone so far as to compare differences in health outcomes between different religious denominations. For example, who has a greater incidence of heart attacks: Catholics or Protestants? Or, how do Jews compare to Christians in survival after being diagnosed with cancer? These studies, comparing the influence of religious denominations on recovery, are the next logical step in the research that examines the influence of religious practices on health. But what will the end results be? If certain religious denominations are associated with better health, should your doctor recommend that you convert to Christianity to reduce your risk of heart disease? Or that you attend Jewish services so that you can lower your risk of cancer? How would you respond if your doctor told you about this evidence and recommended that you convert to a different religion because that would increase your likelihood of remaining healthy? Should the value of individual religions be determined on the basis of their medical effectiveness?

When I tell people that there's very little evidence linking religious involvement and health, I invariably get the same response: "So what if the evidence is inconclusive? How much harm can it do if doctors encourage their patients to pray or read the Bible or go to church?" In other words, "How can it hurt?"

Each of the preceding cases reveals clearly how it can hurt. Each suggests how serious ethical problems can arise when doctors link religious practices to health. The first case illustrates that attempts to link religion and medicine can have a detrimental effect on the patient being treated. The second case shows that even if certain changes in a patient's lifestyle might be beneficial for health, it may not be the physician's role to suggest these changes if doing so invades the patient's privacy. The third case reveals that the practical implications of scientific research can extend far beyond the boundaries of science. So when people ask, "How much harm can come from doctors' attempts to link religious practice to medicine?" the answer is "Plenty." Ethical violations are serious matters, and even if future studies proved that there was strong evidence linking religious activities to health, we would still need to consider these issues before incorporating religious counseling into the practice of medicine.

## DOING HARM

One of the main principles of biomedical ethics is nonmaleficence, the obligation not to inflict harm on a person. Throughout the history of medicine, "Above all, do no harm" has been a central maxim. This obligation is as old as the Greeks. It is clearly expressed in the Hippocratic oath. Today, the issue of nonmaleficence typically arises in discussions of withholding life-sustaining treatment or administering heroic treatment. For example, a terminally ill patient may request that physicians not engage in cardiopulmonary resuscitation after a heart attack, on the grounds that such heroic treatment will only further extend the patient's suffering. The obligation of nonmaleficence arises because it is unclear which action—providing CPR or withholding it—causes harm. Physicians may not always be able to help patients, but they should never cause harm to come to them. Yet efforts to draw closer relationships between religion and medicine may do just that.

The case of the young woman receiving a diagnosis of cancer illustrates how mixing religion and medicine can cause harm. What was she supposed to say to herself when she learned that she had cancer? That she had been insufficiently faithful? That her religious devotion had flagged and that's why she was sick? It's bad enough to be sick, and worse still to be gravely ill. To add to this the burden or guilt and remorse because of a supposed failure of devotion is unconscionable. But when doctors tell patients that religious activity is good for your health, they also imply the opposite: that failure to remain healthy or failure to recover is due to insufficient religious devotion.

It's easy to imagine how both patients and nonpatients would embrace this view. In 1978, social critic Susan Sontag wrote the brilliant essay "Illness as Metaphor," in which she described how cancer patients were blamed for their illness by ascribing undesirable personality characteristics, e.g., emotional repressiveness, to them. In fact, throughout the history of psychosomatic medicine, we can see example after example of disease conditions being associated with various negative traits. Asthmatics were characterized as overly dependent, hypersensitive, and overly passive. Ulcer patients were seen as maintaining a facade of independence and aggressiveness that concealed insecurity and inferiority. Hypertensive patients were dominated by suppressed anger. Migraine headache patients were overly conscientious and had difficulty handling aggression. More generally, there has been a long and unfortunate tradition of blaming the victims of misfortune. Victims of sexual assaults often complain that they have been blamed for somehow causing their attack. Crime victims often report that they are tacitly accused of having done something that encouraged the crime.

Even in the twenty-first century, we often still confront the age-old folk wisdom that illness is due to our own moral failure. It is not uncommon, even today, to hear patients ask themselves what they did to bring on their disease. For some time now, social psychologists have been interested in this phenomenon. In the 1960s, psychologist Melvin

Lerner began investigating what he referred to as the belief in a just world. According to this belief, people get what they deserve and deserve what they get. From this perspective, the world is a place in which there is a kind of cosmic justice that governs events. People who are good deserve good fates, and people who are bad deserve the opposite. Belief in a just world does not permit events to occur at random. The statement by the father of the young woman whose biopsy was negative is a perfect illustration.

This belief provides a kind of self-protection: if the world is governed by a principle of justice, then each of us should be protected from misfortune because we generally believe that we are good people. Justice demands that good people receive good treatment. But this self-protective view may cause problems when we confront others who appear to be virtuous or innocent but nevertheless are the victims of some misfortune. How, in a world of justice, can we account for apparently innocent victimization?

The just-world hypothesis suggests several strategies to maintain this belief. When confronted with such a situation, our first attempt is to rectify the injustice. In almost all cases, however, we can't do this. We can't make a patient with cancer not have the disease. When we can't rectify the injustice, we attempt to identify something that the person did to bring on the misfortune. We may, for example, be satisfied to discover that the reason a friend's car was stolen was because he carelessly left his keys in the ignition when he parked it at the mall. Justice is restored in this case because we can identify something that the person did to cause his misfortune.

But what about cases in which we cannot identify something that a person did to bring on the misfortune? Under these circumstances, how can we restore our belief in a world governed by justice, a world in which we get what we deserve and deserve what we get?

This last formulation of the belief in a just world provides a suggestion: if we deserve what we get, perhaps the victim is really not so innocent. Perhaps the victim is the kind of person who actually deserves this fate. According to the just-world hypothesis, our strategy for restoring justice when we can't find something that the person did to cause the misfortune is to disparage the person, to say to ourselves that he's the kind of person who deserves this fate.

Notice how perfectly this describes the psychosomatic attributions about patients with ulcers, asthma, hypertension, or cancer. Ulcer patients conceal a sense of insecurity and inferiority. Hypertensive patients suppress anger. Cancer patients are emotionally repressive. By attributing these negative characteristics to patients, by disparaging them, we can restore a sense of justice. The patients are no longer innocent; they possess characteristics that are undesirable and thus deserve a fate commensurate with these traits.

This kind of cognitive rearrangement is self-protective. After all, if an apparently innocent person is nonetheless afflicted with a serious illness, how can we be certain that the same fate won't befall us? It can't, of course, if we believe that the world is a just place and we are good people.

The just-world hypothesis should also apply in the opposite direction: justice demands that people who are the recipients of good fortune deserve it because of their sterling characteristics. We don't have to look very far to find evidence of this, too. My favorite example is the saintly transformation of Diana Spencer when she married Prince Charles and became Princess Diana. Up to that point, she was a perfectly ordinary rich young woman. But after the good fortune of marrying the heir to the English throne, she was practically beatified. Overnight, she developed virtues not previously seen.

Belief in a just world may underlie the appeal of believing that religious involvement is associated with better health, since religious devotion is generally considered a virtue. If the world is a just place, the virtuous among us will be protected against misfortune. But the converse of this belief can be harmful. It allows us to ascribe personal failures, religious failures, to people who are sick. And if our own health fails, where does that leave us?

Linking scientific research to measures of moral probity or social worth is a dangerous occupation. Perhaps the most famous example of this kind of research is one we have already covered: the now-discredited eugenics policies based on studies about IQ and immigration conducted at the turn of the twentieth century, which suggested that different ethnic groups showed differing levels of moral probity, intelligence, or other measures of social worth. The eugenics movement held that intelligence and character were related to ethnic origin. Not surprisingly, high levels of intelligence and character were, according to the popular view, more likely to be found in Americans of northern rather than southern European origin, and both of these groups were more likely to possess these characteristics than blacks or Jews. Research studies of the era supported these views. Since then, we have discovered that these studies were seriously flawed, so much so that no conclusions could properly be drawn.

Today, most of us do not hold these views. But the impulse to identify negative personal characteristics with physical or psychological states has not disappeared. It simply finds new outlets—and one such outlet is the position that religious involvement is associated with better health. This view is no less dangerous than its predecessors. Since all of us, whether devout or profane, will ultimately succumb to illness, we should avoid laying the additional burden of guilt for moral failure onto those whose physical health fails before our own.

Another kind of harm that can arise from attempts to link religion and medicine occurs when patients spurn conventional medical care in favor of religious practices. Proponents of closer connections between religion and clinical medicine rarely advocate that patients engage in religious practices to the exclusion of standard medical care. But even if they don't suggest such a course of action, their claims regarding the restorative benefits of religious involvement set the stage for some patients to conclude that they do not need standard medical care because their religious practices will protect them.

An extreme example of the problem of establishing closer links between religious practices and medicine involves support for religious determinism, i.e., because it is God's will that someone is sick, there is no need for conventional medical treatment. The tragic consequences of this stance are illustrated by a case that became famous in both medical and legal circles: the Chad Green case.

> Chad Green was a two-year-old boy with acute lymphocytic leukemia who traveled with his parents to the Boston area from their home in Nebraska in 1977 to seek the most current treatment at the Massachusetts General Hospital (MGH). He began an aggressive regimen of chemotherapy that was thought at the time to have a 50 percent likelihood of cure. Initial successful treatment in the hospital was to be followed by a course of outpatient maintenance chemotherapy. Dr. John Truman, Chad's physician, emphasized to the parents that without the chemotherapy, the leukemia would return and Chad would die.
>
> After four months, Chad experienced a relapse and returned to the hospital. Dr. Truman asked the parents if he had difficulty in following the outpatient treatment regimen. They replied that in fact they had not been giving Chad the chemotherapy because they were providing dietary therapy instead, and moreover, if it was "God's will" that the boy die, then that is what should happen. Backed by the enormous resources and reputation of MGH, Chad's physicians sought court action to require that he receive treatment over the objections of his parents on the grounds that Chad's rights to life superseded his parents' rights to decide. Eventually, after various court proceedings, the physicians prevailed, and Chad's medical custody was assigned to the Massachusetts Department of Public Welfare so that he could continue to receive the potentially lifesaving chemotherapy.
>
> One week after a January 1979 court decision against the parents' wish to use the discredited alternative remedy laetrile in his

*treatment program, the Greens left Boston for Mexico, against a*
*court order. There, Chad was treated with intermittent chemother-*
*apy plus laetrile until August 1979. At that time, the parents termi-*
*nated the chemotherapy. Chad died from a relapse of his leukemia*
*on October 12, 1979.*

Of course none of the proponents of bringing religious practices
into clinical medicine would endorse this behavior on the part of
Chad's parents. They would recommend continuing with conventional
medical care *along with* engaging in religious activities. But their enthusiastic endorsement of the health benefits of religious involvement
is likely to have unintended but perfectly foreseeable consequences:
some patients (or parents of patients) will conclude that religious activity itself is sufficient to treat or prevent disease. A recent study, conducted by McCaffrey and colleagues, demonstrated that about 25 to
30 percent of patients who used prayer for chronic conditions or cancer *were not seeing a physician.* For patients with psychiatric conditions,
90 percent of those using prayer were not seeing a mental health
provider. Presumably, they relied solely on prayer because they thought
it was sufficient to treat the condition and no conventional medical
care was required. The results of this decision to rely on religious activities alone for treatment are tragically predictable.

## PRIVACY

The second example presented in the beginning of this chapter addresses the issue of privacy and the limits of medical intervention.
That example was about a doctor recommending a change in marital
status because the evidence showed that married women and men live
longer than their unmarried counterparts. Most of us would reject that
advice because we believe that our decisions about whether we marry
or not are personal and out of bounds for medicine, even if we agree

that marital status is associated with longevity. For many patients, religious pursuits are a private matter, even if the evidence were to show a solid link between religious activity and health.

Should physicians collect information about the religious and spiritual lives of their patients? Some certainly seem to think so. Several influential physicians recommend taking "spiritual histories" from their patients. Of course, physicians routinely collect "histories" from their patients about medical matters. Should they take a history dedicated to spiritual and religious matters?

Dr. Christina Puchalski, the director of the George Washington Institute on Spirituality and Health (GWISH) at George Washington University, recommends that physicians collect a spiritual history from all new patients at the initial intake and annually thereafter. She recommends the following four questions:

1. Do you consider yourself spiritual or religious?
2. How important are these beliefs to you, and do they influence how you care for yourself?
3. Do you belong to a spiritual community?
4. How might health care providers best address any needs in this area?

Dr. Harold Koenig recommends another set of questions:

1. Do your religious or spiritual beliefs provide comfort and support or do they cause stress?
2. How would these beliefs influence your medical decisions if you became sick?
3. Do you have any beliefs that might interfere or conflict with your medical care?
4. Are you a member of a religious or spiritual community and is it supportive?
5. Do you have any spiritual needs that someone should address?

There is something peculiar about these questions. What is the justification for them? Why should physicians ask a set of questions specifically about religion and spirituality? Why not about sports? Why not about music? What about money? After all, we all have a great many interests that are important to us. Why should doctors ask specifically about religion and spirituality but not about these other areas?

Puchalski and Koenig could argue that there is a mass of empirical evidence linking religion and spirituality to beneficial health outcomes. As we saw in Chapter 7, this evidence is not nearly as strong as they suggest, but even if it were, there is also considerable evidence linking other aspects of our lives to better (or worse) health. There is nothing particular about religion or spirituality that justifies a *dedicated* history.

Puchalski and Koenig could also argue that religion and spirituality are important aspects in the lives of many of their patients, so physicians should ask these questions. It certainly is true that for many patients, religion and spirituality are important, but there are a great many other areas of our lives that are also important: family, friends, work, hobbies, etc. For example, for an enormous number of men in America (and an increasingly large number of women), sports are extremely important. Not only do they provide participants with physical activity which may have positive effects on their fitness and health, or present them with additional risks (as in the case of a patient who participates in extreme sports like snowboarding or skydiving), but they also affect a patient's psychological outlook. This point is underscored by a comment made to me by a representative of a religious broadcasting company. He told me that in North Carolina, where he lived, NASCAR was practically a spiritual experience for most people. But no one suggests that physicians collect a dedicated history on sports. Indeed, as Dr. Neil Scheurich of the University of Kentucky has written, we should regard religious values as one of the many important values that patients may hold.

A great many important factors in our lives are associated with health outcomes, but we generally don't believe that they should be discussed in a medical context. We've already considered the association of marital status and health. Socioeconomic status also is associated with health outcomes. That is, people higher on the socioeconomic ladder are healthier than those lower on the ladder. This is one of the most widely recognized facts in biomedicine. But does this justify a doctor recommending to a patient that he earn more money because that would raise his position on the socioeconomic status ladder and reduce his risk of disease? Evidence also suggests that for women, early rather than late childbearing may reduce the risk of various cancers. Should a physician advise a young woman, either married or single, that she should have a child early in life to reduce this risk? To all these questions, most of us would answer with a resounding "no!"

Why do we respond in this way? Why do we find it objectionable for a physician to make such recommendations? Because we regard these matters as personal and private, even if evidence shows that they are associated with health outcomes. Many patients regard their religious faith as even more personal and private. Not everything that is associated with health outcomes is appropriate for physician inquiries and recommendations. Some matters, regardless of their link to health, are out of bounds for physicians.

Proponents of linking religion and medicine dismiss this argument, asserting that many activities previously considered private and personal, e.g., sexuality, are now routine matters for discussions with physicians. While this is true, the links between aspects of sexuality and health are much stronger than those between religion and health. We know of a great many sexually transmitted diseases, some of which, like AIDS, are potentially fatal. There are no religiously transmitted diseases. Sexuality is a biological function. Religion is not.

Moreover, there are qualitative differences between sexuality and religion. Sexuality, an important and pleasurable aspect of human existence, is not in the same category as concerns about transcendence and meaning. My colleague Catholic chaplain Margot Hover, of Barnes-Jewish Hospital in St. Louis, commented that for many patients, religious concerns are much more freighted than sexual ones. A person's relationship with a divine presence, regardless of religious denominational affiliation, is of a different nature than concerns about sexual matters. To equate the two in the service of bringing religion into medicine is to trivialize religion, a topic we will come to soon.

Collecting a *dedicated* history about religion and spirituality implies a degree of importance based on the physician's values, not necessarily the patient's. This is illustrated by a recommendation by Matthews et al., that clinicians ask, "What can I do to support your faith or religious commitment?" to patients who respond favorably to questions about whether religion or faith are "helpful in handling your illness." We may quite reasonably ask, why is this the business of the physician? Continuing with the example from above, sports may be helpful in handling an illness, for example, by providing a pleasurable distraction or because of the generally beneficial effects of exercise. Should physicians ask how they can help support the interest in sports that their patients have?

A safer course of action is to conduct an ordinary history and ask questions about all aspects of a patient's life, especially as they might influence treatment. Doctors should allow the patients to tell them what is important. Physicians should know this information about a patient, as they should know whether a patient is single, a vegetarian, an employee in a dangerous profession, or homosexual. Information of this sort might be relevant to risk of disease or future treatment and so should be noted in the chart. The point is to allow the patient to express those aspects of his or her life that are important and not a priori assume that some things are more important than others. To do otherwise is to use the authority of the doctor to invade the privacy of the patient.

A third ethical problem raised by close relationships between religion and medicine is manipulation and coercion. To understand this completely, we first need to consider briefly the physician-patient relationship.

# PHYSICIAN-PATIENT RELATIONSHIP: SPECIAL EXPECTATIONS, SPECIAL OBLIGATIONS

As patients, we see physicians for the medical expertise they possess, in the same way that taxpayers see tax accountants or attorneys, and homeowners may seek the advice of a construction engineer, for their special expertise. This relationship to an expert brings with it certain expectations and norms. We expect that the expert is a professional, an authority who has specialized training, ability, and experience in the given field. We anticipate that the expert, whether the physician or the accountant or engineer, will make recommendations that the patient or taxpayer or homeowner is expected to follow. As such, this relationship is asymmetrical: one party makes recommendations and the other follows them.

Think about how different this relationship is from the relationships you have with friends or family. Among friends or business partners, no one in particular has power over another. The relationship is based on equality, not expertise. However, the relationship between expert and client is not based on equality. It is based on the experience and special knowledge of the expert, and the asymmetry is limited to the area of the expert's specialization. The willingness of the homeowner, for example, to follow the engineer's advice is restricted to recommendations about construction and building design. We don't expect engineers to make recommendations outside their area of expertise, in medicine or accounting, for example. And we certainly don't expect homeowners to accept an engineer's medical or accounting advice, even if a misguided engineer were to offer it. An engineer has no more expertise in medicine than a homeowner. On these matters outside the area of expertise, a relationship of asymmetry is inappropriate.

When experts attempt to use the authority of their position to offer advice beyond their area of expertise, they violate the accepted norms of their relationship and run the risk of manipulating or even coercing the client. While this problem is unlikely to occur in accounting or engineering, where the lines defining these fields are clearly drawn, the situation is more serious in medicine, where physical health, even life itself, may be at stake. Physicians often see patients who are sick, fearful, in pain, and therefore especially vulnerable to manipulation. The institutional trappings of medicine reinforce the asymmetry of the relationship. The patient *waits* for the physician to see him or her. The physician asks *personal* questions of the patient and *touches* the patient in ways that, in other settings, would be described as intimate. The physician runs *diagnostic tests* on the patient. Patients often *undress and wear a gown* in the consulting room. Of course, the physician remains fully clothed, often wearing a white coat, a symbol of authority.

All of these characteristics reinforce the aura of authority of the physician and the power he or she has in the physician-patient relationship. Nothing of the sort exists in the relationships we have with accountants or engineers. In recognition of the dangers inherent in this asymmetrical relationship, biomedical ethicists have long recognized the importance of respecting the autonomy of patients. Autonomy requires that patients have the capacity to act and to do so independently. To act autonomously, patients must be competent to act in their self-interest. Unconscious patients, for instance, are unable to act in their self-interest. Assuming they are competent, patients must be allowed to make judgments that are free from untoward influence.

This is especially important when it comes to religious freedom, a matter that is both historically and currently significant in the U.S. The continuing debate about the separation of church and state illustrates how religious freedom is an issue of great importance. (We discuss this specific matter below.)

## Manipulation and Coercion

The principle of autonomy holds that patients should be able to act in an informed manner, free from untoward influence, about their medical care. Concerns about autonomy have been raised by ethicists and philosophers since the Greeks, and they remain important today.

Some social theorists have argued that in American society, autonomy is especially important. After all, the American Revolution was fought to free the colonies from the rule of Britain. Enduring tales of the American frontier speak to the desire to be autonomous and in control of one's own fortune. Traditional American conservative political views express these concerns.

Physicians have a moral obligation to respect patient autonomy and to avoid engaging in manipulation or coercion that is made possible by the medical authority they possess. When considering manipulation or coercion, always keep in mind the important specifics of the doctor-patient relationship: that patients are especially vulnerable because they may be sick, afraid, and in pain.

How does this relate to religion and medicine? When physicians make suggestions, whether explicit or implicit, about the health value of religious practices, they violate the norms of the physician-patient relationship because physicians have no greater expertise than patients in religious matters. Correspondingly, they run the risk of using the authority of their position in manipulative or even coercive ways. The same, of course, applies to physicians making recommendations about tax matters or the appropriate construction of a roof.

Most proponents of closer ties between religion and health make it clear that they believe that proselytizing by physicians is inappropriate and unethical. Doctors should never attempt to encourage patients to engage in religious practices that the doctor thinks are appropriate. Doctors should never make medical care contingent upon certain religious beliefs or practices. The degree of outright proselytizing in medicine is unclear, although as we'll soon see, it does exist. But there are different degrees of physician influence on patients, from the very subtle to the outright manipulative or coercive.

Much of the writing of advocates raises concerns about the possibility of manipulation. For example, in *The Healing Power of Faith,*

Dr. Harold Koenig, a psychiatrist, recommends enhancing the health of patients who are not religious by encouraging them to:

- attend a church or synagogue
- read religious scripture
- emulate the behavior of truly religious/spiritual persons at their place of work

He encourages patients who are already religious to:

- attend services more frequently
- attend a prayer or scripture study group weekly
- get up thirty minutes earlier and spend that time in prayer
- take a few minutes each day to pray with your family

These recommendations would be perfectly acceptable if they came from a member of the clergy. But they did not; they were written by a physician who suggests that following them will lead to better health. Their force derives from Dr. Koenig's position as a medical authority, reinforced by the fact that in broadcast and print media appearances, Dr. Koenig has appeared in a white coat and even carries a stethoscope, even though he is a psychiatrist. Trading on the weight of medical authority, these recommendations are manipulative, and they threaten our religious freedom. Patients are perfectly capable of making religious decisions on their own without interference from doctors.

We saw earlier in this chapter that some proponents of bringing religion into clinical medicine recommend conducting a spiritual history. Both Christina Puchalski and Harold Koenig recommend that these histories be conducted in a completely nonevaluative way so as to avoid efforts to influence patients. However, not all physicians believe that attempts to influence are inappropriate. *The Saline Solution* is a publication of the Christian Medical and Dental Association. Its subtitle is "Sharing Christ in a Busy Practice," and its aim is to help physicians develop proficiency in evangelizing in their interactions with their patients. It teaches doctors how to take a spiritual history, make spiritual diagnoses, and give spiritual prescriptions.

Authors Walter Larimore and William Peel write of various "phases" of evangelism in medical practice, beginning with "cultivation" of their patients, then turning to "sowing" and finally to "harvesting." They see the clinical medical interaction as fertile ground for this. "If we could have designed a more ideal environment for the cultivation phase of a person's spiritual journey, I don't know what we would add."

Indeed, *The Saline Solution* is a manual for using the privileged position of doctor to convert patients to Christianity. Doctors are advised to issue probes, called "faith flags," designed to determine how receptive their patients are to escalating efforts at evangelizing. Faith flags should identify the doctor as a person to whom religion, God, and the Bible are important. They should be very brief, not more than thirty seconds, and should occur naturally in the conversation. Here is an example, taken from an article published in *The Saline Solution*.

> *I went to a new physician the other day. . . . During the exam he asked about my family and I said I had a son in seminary. He asked which one and I said Trinity Evangelical Divinity Seminary in Northbrook, and he said "Ravi Zacharias [head of Ravi Zacharias International Ministries and a graduate of Trinity] has meant so much to me. Are you familiar with him?" He was pressed for time . . . so the conversation changed immediately. But you can be sure as the relationship develops we will be talking about this matter. When I left the office it suddenly dawned on me, I had just been FAITH-FLAGGED!*

This new physician quite skillfully planted the seeds of further discussions of religion in this "cultivation" phase of the doctor-patient relationship. Here are some other examples of "faith flags":

*To a patient facing surgery, the doctor asks "do you know any-
one who prays? You may want to consider asking them to pray for
you because the research clearly shows prayer improves surgical
outcomes."*

*"It may not be important to you, but it would mean a lot to me
if you would let me pray for you. Is that OK?"*

Faith flags may be supplemented by "faith stories," the "next communication step beyond faith flags." "A faith story simply portrays in
narrative form how God or a biblical principle became real or relevant
in your life." They should not take more than two minutes and should
fit naturally into the conversation.

According to *The Saline Solution,* this is a faith story that Dr. Larimore has used in his own practice:

*When we were pregnant with our first child, our family doctor
gave me the assignment of praying for my wife and my child every
night. I had never done this before. At first, it was really uncomfort-
able. I thought Barb would laugh at me or something. But she
didn't. We became closer. We couldn't go to sleep mad at each other
anymore because of our prayer time. We have learned over the sixteen years since then that the family that prays together truly does
stay together.*

Here's an even briefer faith story:

*It may surprise you to learn that many of the decisions I make to
manage my medical practice are based on the Bible.*

It's obvious that the objective of this strategy is to evangelize in a
very gradual manner. "Remember that you're not trying to get a person
to pray the prayer. All you are trying to do is get them one step further,

and you can accomplish that with each visit." Doctors receive the following advice:

"Listen for expressions of interest in the area of personal background."

"Listen for expressions of previous religious experience. This will help you avoid land mines as well as give you stepping stones to build on."

"Proceed slowly. Don't get anxious."

"Regulate the dosage. Take one step at a time."

"Be sensitive to your listener."

"Make sure you're personal and not preachy."

"Point out the specific needs or circumstances that made you aware of your need for Christ."

"Don't oversell."

"Avoid pushing for a decision."

The intent of these statements is obvious: they are part of a subtle, very gradual, and comprehensive effort to reel in a "prospect."

Larimore and Peel make it clear that, contrary to the advice of those who recommend conducting a spiritual history, the physician should not be deterred when a patient expresses lack of interest in religious or spiritual matters. In a hypothetical case study, they write the following: "Raising faith flags and telling faith stories over the years has generated several conversations about spiritual things where *she made it clear that she is not interested in spiritual things*. At every mention of a personal relationship with God, she had an objection [emphasis added]." Despite the repeated expression of noninterest, the physician in this case continued to pursue the matter.

In another hypothetical case, they write that "over ten years, Mr. Brennan has heard numerous faith flags, has been informed of the health benefits of faith, and has seen real faith lived out every time he has had a doctor's appointment." Nonetheless, he has resisted the attempts to evangelize; but apparently, that did not stop the efforts.

Still another hypothetical case shows the same attempt to persuade, albeit gently, despite repeated remarks of noninterest. "You know from her history that she has little spiritual background and interest. Neither has she responded to the faith flags you've raised in the past. . . . You decide to take a chance and relate a brief story of how you found peace when you were faced with an illness. . . . You conclude, 'Jan, God didn't heal me immediately like I asked. . . . I'd love to tell you more sometime, if you're interested.'"

In each of these cases, the physician repeats attempts to persuade a patient who is clearly not interested. Note that in all these cases, the doctors don't merely attempt to encourage religiosity in general on the part of the patients. They attempt to encourage *their* religion. This is an unambiguous attempt to manipulate a potentially vulnerable patient.

If the hypothetical doctors in these vignettes advertise themselves clearly as Christian physicians, then there is no ethical objection to this practice of evangelizing in their medical practice, because patients are well informed of their orientation and know what to expect. However, there is no indication in *The Saline Solution* of such warning. There is no disclosure of their aims. Thus, the approach Larimore and Peel describe violates the standards of informed consent.

## Informed Consent and the Protection of the Patient

Informed consent refers to the process that allows fully informed patients to participate in choices about their health care. It arose out of the Nuremberg trials of Nazi war criminals who conducted horrifying medical experiments on prisoners in concentration camps. The aim of obtaining informed consent is to protect the patient or the research subject.

As an ethical standard, it has evolved from its first use in the 1940s. Today, the primary focus of informed-consent procedures is patient autonomy to make medical decisions in a knowledgeable (i.e., informed) and voluntary manner. Patients should be free to choose or reject the medical care they receive.

To act autonomously, of course, patients must receive complete information about the doctor's intentions. Thus, full disclosure is a central element of informed consent. A patient cannot agree to a medical procedure in an informed way if the physician has not fully disclosed all relevant information.

Following the recommendations of *The Saline Solution* is antithetical to full disclosure. Indeed, the entire enterprise of issuing faith flags and then faith stories is to incrementally identify and then begin to "reel in" a prospect without revealing the aim of the physician. And it is achieving the *doctor's* aim, not the patient's, that is the objective of *The Saline Solution*. This is a violation of the ethical standards that govern medical practice in the U.S. What Larimore and Peel present is a program of covert manipulation to pursue the doctor's agenda, not the patient's.

As we discussed above, this behavior would be acceptable if the physician openly announced that he or she practiced Christian medicine and explained to patients what this meant. To satisfy the requirements of informed consent, this explanation would have to reveal that evangelizing was the doctor's aim.

There is another, more subtle ethical violation in the recommendations of *The Saline Solution*. It is possible, perhaps even likely, that by pursuing the aims of evangelism in clinical practice, the physician will be less attentive to the requirements of acceptable medical care. This will vary from physician to physician, but the potential to be distracted by pursuing the cultivation, sowing, and harvesting of patients is real.

In addition to the possibility of harming the patient by providing substandard care, there is the potential for psychological distress. We can easily imagine how patients might be harmed when they discover that they have been deceived by the doctor, who was more interested in his or her goals than those of the patient.

Keep in mind that this criticism does not pertain to Christian evangelism in general, only its use in the very specific context of the doctor-patient relationship, where the physician has great power over the patient. In other settings, when the two people are on equal footing, the recipient of the evangelical message is free to accept or reject it. Patients, on the other hand, may be sick, in pain, fearful, and otherwise vulnerable to influence in a way that is not characteristic of other aspects of their lives.

Incidentally, attempts at manipulation may work in the other direction, too. Consider a situation that might occur at any major medical center around the country. A devoutly religious young woman learns that the fetus she is carrying has significant, potentially life-threatening anomalies. At a minimum, if the pregnancy goes to term, the infant will be seriously deformed, live a short, painful life, and then die. The woman's obstetrician encourages her to terminate the pregnancy, but the patient refuses on religious grounds. Nevertheless, the physician continues to attempt to persuade her to go ahead with the abortion. Here we have another case in which a doctor attempts to influence a patient to behave in a way inconsistent with her religious convictions. So the concern about manipulation is not always about influencing a patient to adopt new and additional religious habits. It can just as easily be about pressing patients to abandon existing religious convictions.

Another example of a highly questionable attempt to exert influence over a vulnerable patient is the one we encountered at the very beginning of the book: the case of the Colorado orthopedic surgeon shown on the CBS Sunday Morning news program broadcast on February 22, 2004. As the program shows, this surgeon "asks" patients to pray with him when they are gowned and lying on the gurney ready to go into the operating room. This is not mere manipulation. It is outright coercion. Would you feel free to deny this request to pray with a physician dressed in surgical scrubs who is about to have your medical future in his hands, who is about to take a scalpel to your body?

Not very likely. More likely, the "request" will be experienced as an implicit demand from the doctor. But what if you are not particularly religious and you are confronted with such a request. Would you feel free to disagree with the doctor? What if you were deeply religious but believed only in prayers of praise, not prayers of petition, as some of my Jesuit colleagues do? That is, what if you didn't believe in using prayer to *ask for something* but, rather, believed that prayer should be offered only in praise? Would you want to engage in this conversation at this time with this physician, who is about to operate on you? Clearly, the patient's freedom of religious expression is threatened by the surgeon's actions.

Let's take a step back and look at this issue from a broader perspective. How free do patients feel, in less extreme situations, to disagree with physicians' recommendations? How comfortable do patients feel to question their doctor's expertise? Consider the experience of receiving a medical diagnosis and seeking a second opinion about the diagnosis or treatment options. It is standard practice to seek second (and sometimes third) opinions these days when a difficult medical procedure is contemplated. But how comfortable are you with telling your physician that you want a second opinion? Are you concerned that the physician will take this request as a slight, as a criticism, as an implicit rebuke? That as a result of your request, you will not receive the same level of care? That as a result, the physician will not devote the same degree of attention to you? Challenging the recommendations of physicians is difficult for most people. A recent study about prostate cancer treatment revealed that patients feared appearing disrespectful to their doctors by challenging their decisions. Even medical professionals, when in the role of patient, have these concerns.

Why do we care if physicians engage in potentially manipulative efforts to encourage patients to engage in religious activities? How can it hurt? It can hurt because it presents a threat to religious freedom—and religious freedom is a value of great importance in the U.S. One of the founding ideals of the United States was freedom of worship. Freedom to practice religion as you see fit is a great civic virtue, and we frown on activities that threaten to manipulate our practice of religion.

The First Amendment of the Constitution bans the establishment of an official religion in the country. For decades, constitutional scholars have debated precisely what this means, and while the details of this debate are not directly important for us, it is generally relevant to concerns about coercion and manipulation in the medical interaction. Freedom to practice religion without interference benefits both individuals and religion itself.

The conventional view of the ban on establishing an official religion in the U.S. is that it protects government from the influence of religion. However, some historians, for example, Garry Wills, contend that the ban on establishment of an official religion was implemented not to protect the government from religion but rather *to protect religion from the influence of government*. James Madison, even more than Thomas Jefferson, opposed the establishment of an official state religion, because he believed that "religion flourishes in greater purity without than with the aid of government." According to Wills, Madison and Jefferson believed that "churches freed from the compromises of establishment [i.e., of links to government] would have greater moral force."

Thus, government coercion of religious practice is prohibited in the U.S. because it is bad for individual citizens and because it is bad for religion. Coercive pressure, whether from a school system or a physician, to behave in specific ways religiously inhibits the free expression of religious pursuits. Similarly, encouraging the practice of religious activities in the service of better health has the potential to be manipulative or even coercive in a medical interaction between a vulnerable patient and a medical authority. When physicians take on the work of the clergy, they become both bad clergy and bad doctors.

## WHAT CONCLUSIONS CAN WE DRAW?

We began this chapter by asking how it could hurt for doctors to bring religious considerations into the practice of clinical medicine. As we have seen, there are a great many ways in which it can hurt. Physicians run the risk of engaging in manipulative or even coercive actions that threaten the religious freedom of their patients. By probing the religious beliefs of patients, they can invade their privacy. And there is a risk of actually causing harm to a patient who is already vulnerable. By encouraging the belief that religious activities can promote health, doctors risk some patients concluding that they can dispense with conventional medical care in favor of religious practices.

These risks should make us very cautious indeed about introducing religious practices into clinical medicine even if more rigorous future studies should support that there is a connection. Of course, patients may already rely on religious practices to bring them comfort when medical problems arise, unrelated to any effort on the part of the physician to encourage them. If this is the case, then the risk of harm is greatly (though not entirely) reduced. Patients can and should use their religious practices as they always have, without interference from doctors. The dangers arise when the doctor's prestige and power in the physician-patient relationship is used to promote religious pursuits. When this occurs, the doctor violates the most basic maxim of medicine: Above all else, do no harm.

# 11

## IS IT PRACTICAL TO BRING RELIGION
## INTO MEDICINE?

**With so many people asking that religion be brought** into the practice of medicine, it would seem to be a simple thing to do. In fact, though, there are any number of purely practical reasons why it is far more difficult than it appears. One difficulty has to do with the role we expect physicians to play in relation to their patients. Another is the limited amount of time that physicians have to spend with patients. A third problem is whether the training that doctors receive and the expertise they possess allow them to adequately address religious and spiritual matters.

## TAKING A PATIENT'S SPIRITUAL HISTORY    THE ROLE OF THE PHYSICIAN

Everyone recognizes that it is critical for physicians to learn important information about their patients. The Association of American Medical Colleges' Medical School Objectives Project states that physicians "must seek to understand the meaning of the patients' stories in the contexts of the patients' beliefs, and family and cultural values. They must avoid being judgmental when the patients' beliefs and values conflict with their own." Views on religion and spirituality are among the many important matters that physicians must learn about their patients.

We saw in the previous chapter how several prominent physicians recommend conducting "spiritual histories" of their patients, in much the same way that they conduct medical histories. In that chapter, we considered the ethical concerns associated with taking spiritual histories. Here, we consider some of the more practical issues that they raise.

Dr. Christina Puchalski of the George Washington Institute on Spirituality and Health is one of many doctors who favor taking a spiritual history. She has assumed a leading role in promoting the practice. Other doctors, too, recommend conducting spiritual histories, some of which are considerably more extensive and time-consuming. While the questions in these religious/spiritual histories differ in some respects, they share a great deal in common. One essential characteristic, according to virtually all who recommend them, is that they be conducted in a supportive and nonjudgmental manner, consistent with the aims of the Medical School Objectives Project. By so doing, the physician can encourage the patient to use the identified religious or spiritual practices and beliefs as resources for coping with illness or recovery without fear of disapproval by the doctor.

Koenig provides an illustration of this nonjudgmental approach. In a case presentation of an elderly woman with chronic pain and strong religious beliefs, he endorses the woman's assertion that her religious rituals have helped her cope with her pain and encourages her to continue to use religion in this way. "Keep it up!" he says.

On the surface, Koenig's response seems natural and appropriate. Certainly, he believes her religious rituals truly are ways for her to manage her pain. But, as the exploration below will suggest, there is another reason for his enthusiastic endorsement. Dr. Koenig *approves* of her approach to pain management. And his approval raises some very thorny issues. What if he *didn't* approve?

Let's have some fun and rewrite the case Dr. Koenig presents.

*A young woman with Crohn's disease, a serious gastrointestinal disorder, tells Dr. Koenig that she copes with the pain and discomfort of her disease by regularly meeting with her girlfriends to gossip. Would Dr. Koenig say, "Keep it up"?*

*A young man with crippling and painful rheumatoid arthritis reports that he copes with the pain of his illness by watching pornographic videos and reading porno magazines. Would Dr. Koenig say, "Keep it up"?*

*A middle-aged man going through a grueling chemotherapy treatment informs the good Dr. Koenig that it is his membership in the Aryan Nations organization that gives meaning to his life and allows him to cope with all the side effects of the chemotherapy. Does Dr. Koenig still say, "Keep it up"?*

What would Dr. Koenig do in these three cases? How do they differ from the case of the elderly woman with pain? On one level, they are quite similar to Dr. Koenig's case: in all four, the patient engages in an activity—religious ritual, gossip, pornography, membership in a neo-Nazi group—that manages the pain and discomfort. What distinguishes the cases is not their effectiveness but rather their social acceptability. Religious rituals are held in high esteem in the U.S. today. Gossip has relatively little redeeming social value but is generally harmless. On the other hand, watching pornographic videos is socially censured even if it is common. And being a member of a neo-Nazi organization is vilified.

But even membership in hate groups may have beneficial health effects. As sociologist Nancy Rosenblum has observed, groups like the Posse Comitatus and Christian Identity Movement offer many of the characteristics of social connectedness that have been linked repeatedly to health benefits: shared aims, regular meetings, group activities, sense of community, and a common mind-set. Engaging in common acts of resistance like protesting taxation or refusing to appear in courts of law function to bind members socially.

So what will Dr. Koenig, or any other doctor, say to these hypothetical patients who have devised successful, if reprehensible, means to treat their pain? If he says, "Keep it up," is he endorsing these socially vile behaviors and attitudes? If he says nothing or condemns these activities, is he imposing his judgment on his patient? What should he do?

According to the Medical School Objectives Project, there is a clear answer to this dilemma: the physician is supposed to remain nonjudgmental. Despite disapproving of at least some of these successful pain-management strategies, Dr. Koenig nonetheless is obligated by these standards to say, "Keep it up!"

Nevertheless, some of the physicians who support conducting spiritual histories advise distinguishing good forms of coping—religious and otherwise—from ones they consider dysfunctional. Christina Puchalski herself has written that "by inquiring about a patient's beliefs, the physician can assess whether the beliefs are helpful or harmful to the patient's health and medical care." Other proponents of the spiritual history feel the same way. "Physicians need, however, to explore the patient's beliefs, often one-on-one, . . . to be sure that the patient actually subscribes to the relevant tenets of the religion." Whether we agree with this position or not, it's clear that it opposes an entirely nonjudgmental stance and encourages the physician to evaluate the religious or spiritual views the patient has. And as the latter quote directly suggests, the doctor is expected to have sufficient expertise in religion and spirituality to understand "the relevant tenets of the religion."

According to these views, the physician is charged with the responsibility of identifying the dysfunctional religious and spiritual activities and beliefs that patients may have and then correcting them, presumably in the interest of the patient's medical well-being. In more mundane medical matters, this responsibility to correct errors may be appropriate.

Patients may have mistaken beliefs about taking antibiotics, when to take certain medicines, what constitutes sufficient exercise, whether pain is a signal to avoid a certain movement. In such cases, physicians have the expertise to correct these misapprehensions.

But on what basis can they correct religious or spiritual misapprehensions? What qualifies them to do this? Is it even appropriate for them to do so, if they are being nonjudgmental as the guidelines suggest? Assuming this responsibility makes the physician an arbiter of value and meaning in the life of the patient, determining which beliefs and practices are correct and which are not. Do we want physicians to have the power to make these determinations about our religious beliefs? Do *they* want this responsibility?

Even in relatively simple cases, this may not be easy. Most of us would agree that a patient's belief that she is sick because it is God's will is not conducive to coping successfully with the illness. Most would agree that this belief should be addressed and corrected. But on what basis would we correct it? Certainly not on the basis of our knowledge of God's purpose, which we cannot know. The only possible basis for challenging this belief is that *our* reading of religious doctrine differs from the patient's. Why should a physician's view of religious doctrine take priority over the patient's? When did physicians become experts in religious matters?

Thus, the spiritual history raises complexities that are difficult to resolve. To illustrate further, consider the following hypothetical responses to questions posed during a spiritual history. They are an extension of the hypothetical cases of successful pain management above.

Q: What gives your life meaning?
A: *Making as much money as I possibly can.*

Q: Do you belong to a spiritual community?
A: *Yes, I am a member of the Ku Klux Klan.*

Q: Do you consider yourself spiritual or religious?

A: *Yes indeed, I believe in Heaven's Gate and am planning to leave the Earth and board the flying saucer trailing the Hale-Bopp comet.*

Q: What helps you cope with the pain of your condition?

A: *Heroin. It also enhances my spiritual experiences.*

Q: Do you consider yourself spiritual or religious?

A: *No. I used to be but gave it up.*

While these are hypothetical responses and some of them may be extreme, they nonetheless illustrate the dilemma confronting physicians who, according to their own recommendations, must determine whether spiritual and religious beliefs are functional or dysfunctional and then intervene to correct the latter. The physician is assigned the astonishing task of making value judgments about patients' religious and spiritual beliefs. How are physicians to make distinctions between good and bad spiritual beliefs? What qualifies them (addressing the last answer above) to become interpreters and evaluators of the patient's spiritual trajectory from being religious to abandoning it, as some recommend? Astonishingly, some doctors actually believe that they should explore with patients why they have lost their faith and whether there was a good reason for it.

There is absolutely nothing in our understanding of the role played by physicians to suggest that they can function as spiritual guides for their patients, making determinations about what are appropriate and inappropriate religious and spiritual beliefs and actions. Physicians are not guides to the universe's mysteries. Traditionally, we reserve these responsibilities for the clergy.

Dr. Walter Larimore of Focus on the Family, along with two colleagues, attempts to provide some guidance here, endorsing what they call "positive spirituality," which "involves a developing and internalized personal relationship with the sacred or transcendent." Positive spirituality, to be encouraged by the physician, is characterized by "honesty, self-control, love, joy, peace, hope, patience, generosity, forgiveness, thankfulness, kindness, gentleness, goodness, faithfulness, understanding, and compassion" as means toward better mental and physical health. Dysfunctional beliefs are those such as hypocrisy and self-righteousness "that separate people from the community and family, that encourage unquestioning devotion and obedience to a single charismatic leader, or that promote religion or spiritual traditions as a healing practice to the total exclusion of research-based medical care are likely to adversely affect health over time." We might add hubris to this list. But of course, in supporting positive spirituality and discouraging dysfunctional spirituality, physicians must make judgments about what beliefs they consider appropriate.

Larimore, by recommending "positive spirituality" as he defines it, is essentially arguing for patients to be good people. Two questions arise: (1) Is this the job of the physician? and (2) do we have evidence that being a good person as described actually is beneficial for your health?

## IS IT THE PHYSICIAN'S JOB TO PROMOTE THE GOOD? IS BEING A GOOD PERSON GOOD FOR YOUR HEALTH?

Here as elsewhere, we see an expansion of the role of the physician to be a promoter of good, socially desirable behavior. We all know that we should be good people—we should be honest, loving, gentle, and compassionate. Direction such as this typically and appropriately has come from religion and the clergy. Do we need it from physicians? By recommending "positive spirituality," Larimore makes it clear that he imagines the role of the physician to overlap substantially with the role of the clergy.

Even with this guidance, the task of distinguishing good from bad spiritual beliefs is daunting. Larimore and his colleagues recommend censuring "unquestioning devotion and obedience to a single charismatic leader." Where, precisely, does Catholicism fall in this regard? What about the Lubavitcher Jews? Christianity or Islam in general? Don't they encourage unquestioning devotion and obedience to a single charismatic leader? And if it is okay to follow the pope, why is it unacceptable to follow L. Ron Hubbard? Or David Koresh? Or Marshall Applewhite, leader of the Heaven's Gate cult? Is the physician able to make such distinctions and then make recommendations to patients? Would any physician want to?

In 1986, the controversial epidemiologist Petr Skrabanek published an article on preventive medicine and morality. In it, he assailed the increasingly common attempts to conflate ideology and morality with science, declaring such fusing to be "a social movement dressed up in scientific language." Larimore's litany of virtues is a case in point. Honesty, self-control, love, joy, peace, hope, patience, and generosity are, without a doubt, personal characteristics that we favor, but recommending them is a *moral* matter, not a scientific or medical one.

As usual, H. L. Mencken had something sensible, and biting, to say. "Hygiene is the corruption of medicine by morality. It is impossible to find a hygienist who does not debase his theory of the healthful with a theory of the virtuous. The true aim of medicine is not to make men virtuous; it is to safeguard and rescue them from the consequences of their vices." By "hygiene," Mencken meant public health and medicine.

Skrabanek's and Mencken's comments both resonate loudly in connection with contemporary attempts to conflate the "good" or the virtuous, as some define it, with health. "There are many who wish to believe that premarital sex causes venereal diseases, that homosexuality causes AIDS. . . . This is simply not true; infectious diseases are caused by infectious agents."

Larimore et al. endorse characteristics (e.g., joy, faithfulness) which few would dispute as virtues. We all would like to possess these traits and like our friends and relatives to possess them too. But do we have any evidence that these characteristics are good for our health? And if not, why should physicians be making recommendations about them? Again, we see the expansion of the role of the physician to include many of the responsibilities usually assigned to the clergy.

These views reflect the ancient belief that disease is the product of negative personality characteristics, something we reviewed in Chapter 10. The virtuous among us will be resistant to disease, and those of us with character flaws will suffer illness. It is a view that was held by the Greeks, who believed in a relationship between societal virtues and physical health. It is the view that Susan Sontag devastatingly criticized in her brilliant essay "Illness as Metaphor." It is a view consistent with the belief that good things happen to good people, that people get what they deserve and deserve what they get. It is the view that leads people to feel guilt or remorse when they become ill or fail to recover. If virtues are associated with better health, then poor health must be due to an absence of them. This position has no place in medicine.

So conducting spiritual histories appears to be an unrealistic and spectacularly bad idea. While offered in an apparently innocuous package of recommendations about how to incorporate spiritual and religious concerns into medical encounters, such histories will alter substantially the role of the physician as we know it. They require an expansion of this role that includes becoming the arbiter of appropriate and inappropriate religious and spiritual values, even implying that the physician functions as a guide to understanding the mysteries of the universe. Matters of good and evil, virtue and vice, have long been the domain of religion. But they will become medical matters.

To suggest that they become part of a physician's role is an unrealistic and bold extension of the doctor's responsibilities. Is it the responsibility of a physician to act as a spiritual guide?

These supposedly brief, simple spiritual histories raise problems that are enormously difficult even for professional clergy to address, let alone physicians with little if any training in the area and virtually no time in the office. Asking physicians to become the arbiters of values and meaning, of healthy and unhealthy aspects of religion, guides to the mysteries of the universe, is asking the impossible.

This is bad for patients and it is bad for medicine. It's also bad for religion. Attempting to address these weighty matters in a four-minute spiritual history can be accomplished only by trivializing the religious experience. Focusing only on such positive characteristics as love, peace, joy, and patience, as Larimore and colleagues recommend, essentially whitewashes the great drama of judgment, repentance, forgiveness, and reconciliation that characterizes many religions. It converts religion to a Hallmark card.

## RESOURCE ALLOCATION

In the U.S. in the early twenty-first century, physicians constantly complain that they lack the time required to treat patients adequately. Of course, there are many reasons why they may feel this way: increased paperwork, more phone calls, more diagnostic tests, and a greater number of patients. As a result, physicians have an extremely limited amount of time to spend with patients. Therefore, decisions about how to spend this precious time must be made wisely. It can be spent efficiently, and there is no shortage of established practice standards to provide guidance.

One set of guidelines comes from the U.S. Preventive Services Task Force. According to its Web site (www.ahrq.gov/clinic/uspstfab.htm), the task force is "the leading independent panel of private-sector experts in prevention and primary care. The USPSTF conducts rigorous, impartial assessments of the scientific evidence for the effectiveness of a broad range of clinical preventive services, including screening, counseling, and preventive medications. Its recommendations are considered the 'gold standard' for clinical preventive services."

The USPSTF reviews the medical literature and then makes evidence-based recommendations about which practices have been shown to be effective in reducing disease and which ones haven't. It addresses these general disease categories:

Cancer

Heart and Vascular Diseases

Injury and Violence

Infectious Diseases

Mental Conditions and Substance Abuse

Metabolic, Nutritional, and Endocrine Conditions

Musculoskeletal Disorders

Obstetric and Gynecologic Conditions

Pediatric Conditions

Vision and Hearing Disorders

Here are some examples of the recommendations:

- Breast Cancer: Consistent with the USPSTF screening recommendations, a large study published in late 2005 demonstrated that mammography contributed to a substantial reduction in death from breast cancer between 1975 and 2000.
- High Blood Pressure: The USPSTF found that evidence supports the value of measuring blood pressure to identify adults at increased risk for cardiovascular disease due to high blood pressure and that treating high blood pressure substantially decreases the incidence of cardiovascular disease with few risks.
- Hepatitis B: The USPSTF strongly recommended that pregnant women be screened for hepatitis B virus at their first

prenatal medical visit. However, it found insufficient evidence to support screening the general asymptomatic population.
• Depression: The USPSTF recommended that in primary care settings, adult patients be screened for depression and those patients identified as depressed be treated. It concluded that the benefits of screening outweigh any potential risks.

These USPSTF recommendations provide physicians with guidelines about how they should spend their time with their patients, based on evidence about which practices work and which ones don't. According to a recently published report that studied 2,500 patients, *physicians would need to spend 7.4 hours per day* to provide the services required to comply with the task force recommendations. While this may represent an extreme demand on the time of physicians, it nevertheless makes the point that physicians must use the limited amount of time they have with patients wisely. They do not have time to waste on activities that have not been shown to be effective in preventing and treating disease.

Not surprisingly, physicians have great difficulty in complying with these recommendations. For example, another recent study reported that in community-based primary care practices, Pap smears were administered to only 64 percent of women patients. Pap smears, of course, are the primary preventive test for cervical cancer, but according to this report, more than one-third of women patients did not receive them. Only 47 percent of women had discussions about breast self-exams, and only 39 percent of women over age fifty had a mammogram in the past year. Among men and women over age fifty, fewer than 40 percent had a digital rectal exam in the past year, and fewer still had a fecal occult blood test or sigmoidoscopy. Finally, fewer than 30 percent of men had a PSA test. Overall, the report found that only 3 percent of women and 5 percent of men over the age of fifty had all the recommended cancer screening tests.

What's the point of this study? It addresses how wisely and effectively doctors spend their time with patients. The evidence is abundantly clear that these tests are effective ways of screening for cancer and should be part of the care of every patient over a certain age. Nevertheless, doctors appear to spend their time with patients doing other things. Is this a good idea?

Similar time pressure exists for the care of patients with chronic disease, and not surprisingly, there are recommendations about standards of care for these patients. Another recent study examined the degree of physician compliance with these recommendations. It reported that 3.5 hours per day are required to provide adequate care for patients with the top ten chronic diseases, e.g., heart disease or diabetes, *assuming that the disease is stable and under adequate control.* This is for just ten chronic diseases and only for patients whose disease is stable. Of course, more time is required for managing other patients whose disease is not stable or who have other chronic conditions.

Thus, the most *basic* medical services for disease prevention and treatment of chronic diseases require more time than physicians have in the day. Not surprisingly, doctors fall short of full compliance with these practice guidelines. They lack sufficient time for the most basic preventive medicine practices. They screen for depression, diet and nutrition, exercise, even smoking, far too infrequently. Managing only their well-controlled chronic-disease patients would consume nearly half of the day. In response to these demands, primary-care doctors appear to fall short of what is called for. If this is true, where will doctors find the time to conduct spiritual histories, or to engage in the extended discussions of religion and spirituality that these histories may provoke?

The spiritual history, according to Puchalski, can take only four minutes to conduct. That may seem like a relatively short time, but as a result of taking even four minutes to conduct a spiritual history, what will the physician no longer have time for? A Pap smear? A conversation about depression? About diet and exercise? What will the doctor *not* ask about?

Of course, a physician can, as part of the standard history, ask questions to learn about all of the things that are important to patients, but there is no basis for emphasizing religion and spirituality over other aspects of life. A physician can and should ask "Are you a religious or spiritual person?" or "Do you have any religious or spiritual beliefs or practices that might influence your medical care?" But such a question should be asked about any personal activity or belief that might influence medical care. These questions should be asked along with others about family, job, hobbies, and other elements of our lives. But there is no reason to go beyond this. Conducting a dedicated spiritual history means that other, more pressing medical matters will not be addressed. As we will see in the next chapter, when patients are asked if they want discussions of religion and spirituality if it takes time away from conversations about medical matters, only 10 percent of them say that they do.

## TRAINING OF PHYSICIANS

The U.S. has 125 medical schools, and each year more than sixteen thousand students graduate from them. In the *Handbook of Religion and Health,* Harold Koenig and colleagues write that in 1993, fewer than five schools offered some training in religion and spirituality but that by 2000, at least sixty-five offered such courses. Proponents of closer links between religion and medicine suggest that this represents a substantial accomplishment, in that medical students will receive training in addressing the religious and spiritual needs of their patients.

Even if this estimate is accurate, it sheds little light on what is taught in these courses, how much detail they offer, how much time is devoted to this topic, and when in the medical school curriculum they are offered.

By reporting that at least sixty-five U.S. medical schools offer courses on religion and spirituality, we might assume that they are courses similar to the college courses we have taken. College courses typically are a semester in length and generally allow for a reasonably thorough examination of a subject. If this were the case, it might represent a substantial exposure to the topic of religion and health. Unfortunately, a "course" in religion and health never means a semester-length course in medical school. To understand what it does mean, we need to review briefly the basics of medical education in the U.S.

In the U.S., medical school is four years in length. No two medical schools' curricula are identical, but there are substantial similarities among them. At the Mayo Medical School, for example, most of the first academic year is devoted to basic and clinical science. Students study the endocrine system, the digestive system, the renal system, neuroscience, nutrition, pathology, cell biology, anatomy, molecular genetics, immunology, and other topics. In addition, they take a course called "Growth and Development" and a course called "Continuity of Care." According to information the medical schools themselves provide to the Association of American Medical Colleges, spirituality as a topic is covered in these two courses. These course also cover breast cancer, obesity, disability, healthy aging, psychological factors in heart disease, and the impaired physician, so we have no idea how much time is devoted to religion and spirituality. But since these two courses together are six months in length and in the first academic year at Mayo, and there are a total of forty-two months of first-year courses (many of the courses overlap), it's not hard to imagine that students receive relatively little exposure to religion and spirituality.

At Florida State, there is no coursework in religion and spirituality in year one. In year two, however, students are taught "Health Issues in Medicine" and "Psychosocial Aspects of Medicine." These courses consume twenty-one months out of a total of seventy months of year two coursework. The rest of this year is devoted to microbiology, pathology, immunology, pharmacology, infectious diseases, and physiology. At FSU, there is potentially more exposure to information on religion and spirituality than at Mayo, according to the curriculum data provided by the schools themselves, but we still have no idea what proportion of these courses is allotted to these topics as opposed to other issues. In years three and four, FSU offers no training in religion and spirituality.

Again, there is considerable variation in the medical school curricula around the country, but most time in the first two years is devoted to the physical basis of medicine. Once in the third year, medical students begin their clinical clerkships. These clerkships are hands-on training programs in pediatrics, medicine, surgery, obstetrics and gynecology, neurology, psychiatry, and primary-care medicine. Students spend their third year rotating through these medical services under the guidance of senior physicians on the faculty. As trainees, they see patients in every conceivable specialty.

Finally, in the fourth year, students spend their time in a series of electives in a variety of clinical or basic science courses. That is, they can choose how they plan to spend their fourth year, subject to a few general requirements.

So when articles report that over one-half of U.S. medical schools now offer "courses" in religion and health, keep in mind that at best, only a small fraction of coursework may be devoted to this topic. The "course" in religion and spirituality is not the equivalent of other courses we have taken. Exposure to such a "course" hardly qualifies the physician to do anything more than determine if religion and spirituality are important to the patient.

But even this may exaggerate the potential impact of these "courses," since virtually all medical students go on to some form of postgraduate training. This postgraduate education consists of internships (one year), residency programs (two to three years), and fellowships in specialties like orthopedic surgery or psychiatry (three to five years). With the possible exception of postgraduate training in family medicine, it is highly unlikely that there is any further exposure to religion and spirituality.

Only after this training are physicians ready to practice medicine. So by the time the newly trained doctor begins to practice on his or her own, it may be seven or eight years since he or she took one of these "courses" in religion and health offered in the first two years of medical school. Essentially, this is no training at all, certainly not enough to qualify the physician as an expert in this area. The physician has no more expertise than the patient.

So it is reasonable to ask how well prepared for addressing matters of religion and spirituality physicians are with at most only a few hours of training in religion and spirituality they received many years ago in medical school. To answer this question, let's consider the kinds of religious and spiritual concerns that arise in the practice of medicine.

*The patient was a frail, elderly woman, hospitalized with multiple medical problems. Her husband was in the hospital room with her. She complained of being restless and not at peace, and her husband readily agreed, but neither one could shed any additional light on the matter. Consistent with her description, the patient appeared to be tense. She repeatedly commented how good her husband was to her and how committed to their marriage he was. She reported that they had had many years of happy marriage. During this time, the husband appeared to become testy that the conversation was not resolving anything. Eventually, the patient revealed that upon marrying her husband, she had converted to Judaism to meet the expectations of her Orthodox in-laws. Despite keeping a kosher home and complying with some Jewish practices, the patient would often sneak her sons out of the home to attend Christian holiday services. The husband, for his part, was not a practicing Jew. In the patient's later years, after her in-laws had died and her children had grown, she began attending a local Christian church for social activities and then worship. Her husband refused to accompany her, though he himself did not attend any religious services of any kind, Jewish or otherwise. She resented this deeply, considering that she had gone so far as to convert to Judaism when they married, and felt that it was his turn. She confessed that, in fact, she deeply regretted her conversion so many years before. This was the first time she had ever*

*expressed these feelings to her husband. She understood her conver-*
*sion as a betrayal of her Christian faith and a heavy lifelong burden.*

This case illustrates many of the problems confronted by physicians who attempt to address the religious and spiritual concerns of their patients. Note that the issues here were not medical at all. They were interpersonal, marital, and religious. Addressing them adequately requires the skills of a psychotherapist or a pastoral counselor, not a physician. How will a busy physician have the time or experience to address these matters?

I have changed some key details from this case to protect patient privacy. One of the most important details you don't have was that it took nearly an hour to work through these matters. Considering the nature of the problem and the fact that it had persisted for decades, this is not surprising. If you are wondering what kind of a physician has the time or temperament to spend an hour with a patient and her husband to listen to these problems, you are right to wonder. In fact, it wasn't a doctor at all. It was a health care chaplain.

And that's the point. No physician has either the time or the skill to address this kind of a religious or spiritual matter. The problem that this patient had lived with for years involved an intricate web of interpersonal relationships and religious concerns. The former involved her husband, of course. In addition, her husband's parents were involved. And so were her children. And in addition to these overt interpersonal matters, there were covert ones: she hid the fact that she attended Christian holiday services, raising the issue of duplicity in her relationship with her husband and, most likely, her in-laws.

The religious and spiritual matters were at least as complex. She renounced her Christian heritage, the heritage of her family (this is another element of the interpersonal web). She embraced a new religion, Orthodox Judaism. She followed new and unfamiliar religious practices, including keeping a kosher kitchen and other Jewish practices. Added to the mix was the fact that despite the conversion and the Jewish rituals, she nonetheless would contrive to attend Christian holiday services with her sons.

The first question in Dr. Harold Koenig's spiritual history is "Do your religious or spiritual beliefs provide comfort and support or do they cause stress?" If Dr. Koenig had been this patient's doctor and had asked her this question along with the rest of the spiritual history, how would she have responded, and what would Dr. Koenig have done? At least Koenig is a psychiatrist and, presumably, could understand the interpersonal complexities of this case. But what would he have done about the religious and spiritual concerns expressed? And would he have had the time to spend an hour with this patient and her husband in the hospital room? Not likely. Proponents of conducting a spiritual history always mention that it takes only a few minutes to administer. It may be true that it takes only a few minutes to *ask the questions,* but as this case demonstrates, it takes longer—much longer—to listen to the answers.

Earlier in this chapter, we considered the case of the elderly patient who told Dr. Koenig that her religious rituals helped her manage her pain. Dr. Koenig replied to her, "Keep it up!" thus encouraging her to continue. What advice would Dr. Koenig give to this patient who had abandoned the faith of her family? Would he encourage her to return to her Christian faith? Even asking this question demonstrates how ridiculous it is. How could you possibly address a matter of this complexity in a few moments, even if you had the requisite skills, training, and experience?

Making matters even more complex is the fact that in the early twenty-first century, religious heterogeneity is increasing dramatically in the U.S. We could argue that in times when religious affiliation was more homogeneous, physicians and patients would often share a common faith. If that were the case, at least the doctor could have some degree of familiarity with the patient's religion. That wouldn't give the doctor any more expertise in religion than the patient had, of course, and therefore the doctor still wouldn't be entitled to make recommendations to the patient. But at least he or she might understand that patient's faith.

Recent trends in immigration have made this problem even more acute, as America has become the most religiously diverse country on earth. There now are more Muslim Americans in the U.S. than there are Episcopalians or members of the Presbyterian Church. Immigrant Jews from Russia and Ukraine have created increased diversity within the Jewish community in the U.S. According to religious historian Diana Eck, Los Angeles is the most complex Buddhist city in the world, and the U.S. is now the home of about 4 million Buddhists. Even American Christianity has been transformed by immigration from Latin America, the Philippines, Vietnam, and Haiti. According to a study of three decades of religious identification in the U.S., the fraction of the population identifying as Protestant dropped from 63 percent in 1993 to 52 percent in 2002. At the same time, the number of respondents reporting that they had no religion rose from 9 percent to 14 percent.

Why is this increase in religious diversity important? Because it means that the likelihood of physician and patient sharing the same faith is becoming smaller and smaller. We saw above that the extremely limited amount of time medical students spend in coursework on religion and spirituality gives the doctor no special expertise in these matters. With an increasingly religiously diverse population in the U.S., it becomes even less likely that the doctor will even understand the patient's faith, let alone have any expertise in it.

Consider, by contrast, the training received by the clergy in general and by health care chaplains more specifically. At New York City's Union Theological Seminary, generally regarded as a liberal Protestant institution, candidates for the master of divinity degree are required to take the following during the three-year program:

- Biblical Courses
- Historical Courses
- Theological Courses

- Arts of Ministry Courses
- Field Education
- World Religions Course
- "The City" Courses, about ministries in New York City
- Electives courses

The curriculum at the evangelical Fuller Theological Seminary in Pasadena, California, is no less rigorous. At Fuller, the master of divinity degree requires completion of 144 course units, typically over a three- to four-year period. Students can concentrate in Recovery Ministry; Christian Formation and Discipleship; Cross-Cultural Studies; Multicultural Ministries; Family Pastoral Care and Counseling; Youth, Family, and Culture; Family Life Education; and Worship, Theology, and the Arts. Students take courses in Biblical Languages, Biblical Studies, Church History and Theology, Ministry Studies, and other elective programs.

As rigorous and time consuming as this is, even more training is required for health care chaplaincy. Health care chaplains are clergy who have specific training in medicine and health, and typically, they work in hospitals. Health care chaplaincy is like residency training after completing medical school. You can't complete a residency or fellowship in orthopedic surgery, for example, without first having a medical degree. Although the situation is slightly different, almost all health care chaplains have an advanced degree in the ministry, i.e., are a member of the clergy or a selected layperson with a graduate-level theological degree.

In the three-year training program in divinity, students take graduate courses in basic psychology. As chaplains Thomas O'Connor and Elizabeth Meakes point out, training in health care chaplaincy requires *even more* supervision and clinical work. Those who go on to advanced clinical chaplaincy receive an additional four hundred hours of theologically and psychologically informed supervision, and unofficially, trainers typically are referred to personal psychotherapy.

What's the point of this examination of the training that physicians and clergy receive? It's that physicians essentially receive no training in religion and health, even if they have a few hours of exposure in their first or second year of medical school. They have no special qualifications for engaging in religious discussion with their patients. In fact, they are no more knowledgeable about religious and spiritual matters than their patients.

In contrast, the clergy, *legitimate* experts in matters of religion and spirituality, have at least three years of training. If they specialize in religion and medicine, i.e., health care chaplaincy, they have more training still. These professionals are qualified to explore the religious and theological and spiritual aspects of health and illness with patients. Not only do they have the training, but they are not limited, as physicians are, in the time they can spend with patients. Their expertise entitles them to ask probing questions, explore difficult theological matters, interpret religious doctrine, and challenge patients' misunderstandings about religious and spiritual issues. Moreover, health care chaplains typically have considerable training in psychology that permits them to adequately address the kind of situation presented above.

By virtue of their training and expertise, they can function as legitimate religious experts. In Chapter 10 on ethical concerns, we saw that physicians' lack of expertise in this area raises the problem of manipulation or even coercion. Physicians are legitimately able to make recommendations to patients about medical matters because of their expertise in medicine. Because they lack expertise in religion, they lack legitimacy in this area. Clergy, on the other hand, have extensive experience in religion and so are entitled to make recommendations.

In previous chapters, we have seen that the evidence linking religious involvement and health is, at best, weak and inconclusive. We've also seen that there are significant ethical objections to bringing religious practices into clinical medicine. Now we discover that in addition to these problems, there are significant practical reasons why it is a bad idea to closely link religion and health in the context of medical practice. Doing so distorts the traditional role that the doctor plays in the relationship with the patient. It consumes valuable time in the clinical interaction that should better be spent on matters for which there is evidence of a beneficial effect. And it requires a degree of training and experience that doctors simply don't receive.

# 12

## IS THERE REALLY A DEMAND FOR BRINGING
## RELIGION INTO MEDICINE?

**Advocates for a closer relationship between religion** and medicine typically buttress their arguments in several ways. First, they routinely cite statistics about how religious a country the U.S. is in the early twenty-first century. Second, they cite reports from research studies that suggest that patients would like physicians to engage in discussions of religious and spiritual matters as well as religious rituals (e.g., prayer) with them. And, of course, they cite the studies that claim to show health benefits to the religiously active. We have already examined the quality of the evidence about religious involvement and health benefits and shown how poor it is. How valid are these other two justifications, and how solid is the evidence for them?

## ARE AMERICANS AS RELIGIOUS AS
## THE ADVOCATES INDICATE?

At the beginning of most books on religion and health, the authors roll out the same polling data to demonstrate how deeply religious a country the U.S. is. Here are some examples:

- In the introduction to the *Handbook of Religion and Health,* Dr. Harold Koenig and colleagues write, "In 1994, 96 percent of the population of the United States believed in God or a higher power."
- Dr. Herbert Benson, author of *Timeless Healing,* writes, "According to a 1990 Gallup poll, 95 percent of Americans say they believe in God and 76 percent say they pray on a regular basis."
- In *God, Faith, and Health,* Dr. Jeff Levin writes that "national surveys repeatedly show that about 90 percent of Americans, regardless of age, affiliate themselves with a religion or religious denomination."
- In *The Healing Power of Faith,* Harold Koenig writes that "polls indicate that . . . 90 percent [of Americans] pray" and that 43 percent of Americans regularly attend religious services.

Indeed, there are polling data that suggest that very substantial fractions of Americans are religious. According to the Gallup Poll's Web site (http://brain.gallup.com/content/default.aspx?ci=1690&pg=2), 84 percent of those surveyed in 1965 believed in God. In 1999, it was 86 percent, and in 2004 it was 81 percent. These figures are not quite as high as those cited above but are still quite high. The Web site also indicates that from 1939 to 2005, 37 to 49 percent of those surveyed reported that they attended church or synagogue in the week before they were surveyed. For the period from 1992 to 2005, those who reported that they attended once per week ranged from 28 to 36 percent. For those reporting attendance almost every week, the range was 9 to 14 percent.

The contrast between the U.S. and other Western countries is striking. According to the World Values Survey published in the year 2000, approximately half of those surveyed in western European countries never or practically never attended religious services. For example, in France, 60 percent of those surveyed never or practically never attended services. In the UK, it was 55 percent. In the Netherlands, it was 48 percent. Sweden and Denmark, 46 percent and 43 percent. In the United States, only 16 percent reported that they never or practically never attended religious services.

So there is, in fact, a great deal of survey data to indicate that Americans as a whole are very religious and more so than citizens of other Western countries. However, some evidence suggests that some of these survey data may be upwardly biased, and as a result, the real rates of religious involvement in the U.S. may be lower than these surveys report.

In the examination of the studies of religious attendance and mortality (see Chapter 8), we saw how estimates of attendance at services don't always represent the situation as it exists in the real world, especially when the estimates of attendance are taken from studies that rely on interviews for data collection. Remember what we discovered from these interviews: interpersonal interactions either in person or over the telephone raise concerns about how respondents may appear to the interviewer, thus leading them to overstate their degree of attendance at religious services anywhere from 30 to 50 percent.

This bias also is likely to affect survey reports about other religious characteristics (e.g., belief in a god or spirit) and about the degree of religiosity, too. In these cases, it seems fair to assume that data derived from surveys that use interview methods are affected by the same sort of concerns about self-image that tend to bias attendance data. This is precisely what the Harris Interactive Poll online between September 16 and 23, 2003, showed. The poll, based on a national sample of 2,306 adults, found that 79 percent of Americans reported that they believe there is a God. This percentage is substantially lower than the results of Gallup Polls cited by the authors above. According to the Harris Poll no. 59, October 15, 2003 (www.harrisinteractive.com/harris_poll/index.asp?PID=408), the lower results are due to the fact that when data are collected online, they are not subject to the self-presentation biases that affect how people describe themselves when they are being interviewed face-to-face or over the phone. Like the religious-attendance data, these results regarding people's belief in God are likely to be overstated by a considerable margin.

Other data also call into question the estimates of the great religiosity in the U.S., and of course these data also are not presented by advocates. Gallup surveys over the last thirty years of the twentieth century showed remarkable stability in responses to questions about whether respondents attended religious services in the seven days prior to being surveyed: approximately 40 percent of respondents indicated that they had. In contrast, time-use data tell a very different story. Remember that unlike surveys that collect data by interviews specifically asking about the issue in question, time-use surveys ask only about what participants did at a specific time on a specific day. According to sociologists Stanley Presser and Linda Stinson, the time-use data indicate that religious attendance dropped by about 30 percent between 1966 and 1975 and then dropped an additional 5 percent from 1975 to 1994. Their data suggest that attendance was not stable at all.

This doesn't mean that there is no evidence whatsoever about the religiosity of Americans. Even the less biased Harris survey still showed that four-fifths of respondents reported believing in God. Even the data from time-use surveys that do not rely on interview methods indicate that about 25 percent of those surveyed attended religious services regularly. However, these rates of religiosity are not as astronomically high as those reported in the many books on religion and health. And the high level of belief in God does not appear to translate into an equally high rate of attendance at religious services.

It's also important to look at this issue from a different angle and ask a provocative question: Isn't there something peculiar about citing the high level of religiosity in America as a justification for bringing religion into medical practice? Even if the surveys are correct about the level of religiosity, does that really mean that people necessarily want to link religion to medicine? Do people really want their doctors treating them with prayers along with Prozac? When the chips are down, do Americans afflicted with cancer really want a dose of the Ten Commandments in addition to state-of-the-art chemotherapy? The great Supreme Court justice William Brennan was a devout Catholic who attended mass every day. But he believed that his religious devotion was a private matter that was not to be introduced into other aspects of his life. People can value religion profoundly but still regard it as separate from other realms of their lives.

## DO PATIENTS WANT CLOSER LINKS BETWEEN RELIGION AND HEALTH?

Advocates also like to cite studies demonstrating that patients want closer links between religion and medicine. Studies do, in fact, report that some patients want their physicians to attend to their spiritual concerns. For example, researchers Dana King and Bruce Bushwick interviewed 203 hospitalized patients from family practices about their views on the relationship between religion and health. Over three-fourths said that doctors should consider patients' spiritual needs, and 37 percent wanted more frequent discussions of their religious beliefs with physicians. Forty-eight percent reported that they wanted their doctors to pray with them. Drs. Todd Maugans and William Wadland reported that 40 percent of their patients wanted their physicians to discuss religious issues with them. Timothy Daaleman and Donald Nease found that 63 percent of patients who regularly attended religious services believed that physicians should ask about religious and personal faith. On the other hand, only 13 percent of patients who attended services only infrequently wanted doctors to inquire about religion.

These data have prompted some to remark that regardless of the evidence about relationships between religion and health, "we should address [religion in medical practice] because the patient surveys are saying that we should be addressing it."

Is that really true? Are they really saying that? In none of the three studies cited above did a majority of all patients report that they approved of having physicians ask questions about religion and spirituality in the context of a family practice setting. The claims that patients are asking physicians to address religious and spiritual questions are even further qualified.

For example, the King and Bushwick study is often cited as indicating patient interest in bringing religion into clinical medicine. In the study, 37 percent of the respondents reported that they felt their physicians should discuss religious matters more; however, the paper contains other relevant information. There is, most important, a very interesting result never trumpeted by those hoping to bring religion into the doctor's office: *47 percent of the patients reported that they wanted no discussion at all* and another 3 percent reported they wanted less discussion. This important fact is not even reported in the paper. You have to compute it yourself from one of the tables. That is, half of the patients wanted less discussion or none at all. It's not even in the paper's abstract, which presented only the information on those 37 percent who wanted discussions of religious matters with their physicians. So the King and Bushwick study provides little evidence of an overwhelming desire on the part of patients for greater involvement of religion in medical practice. In fact, it presents data that suggest the opposite: patients want less talk about religion from their doctors.

In another study, John Ehman et al. reported that about two-thirds of the patients they questioned approved of physician inquiries into religious and spiritual matters. However, in this study, patients were not asked about this matter in general but specifically if such physician inquiries would be acceptable to them *if they became gravely ill*. It's easy to imagine that people who are gravely ill will turn their minds toward spiritual concerns. This should surprise no one who has watched a relative or friend die of a terminal illness. Religion frequently plays a role at the end of one's life, but this study then tells us nothing about whether the great majority of patients who are *not* gravely ill would find it acceptable. There are other studies, however, that do look at patients in different stages of illness and health.

For example, Christopher Mansfield and colleagues reported the results of a survey of 1,033 randomly selected adults in eastern North Carolina. The location is important because this is in the Bible Belt, a part of the country in which belief in God and attendance at religious services is especially high. This study is the only report on the demand of patients for discussing religious and spiritual matters with their physicians that is based on a randomly generated sample. According to this report, over two-thirds of the respondents reported that they probably would or definitely would want to talk to someone about spiritual concerns if they were seriously ill or injured badly enough to be hospitalized. However, *only 2 percent said that their first choice for such a person to speak to would be a physician.* Overwhelmingly, their first choice was a minister. Only 1 percent included a physician as one of multiple people they would choose to speak to. If, in the Bible Belt, patients have so little interest in involving a doctor in discussions of spiritual concerns about serious illness or injury, how high can it be in other parts of the country where interest in religion is much lower?

In a much more geographically representative study, 456 patients from primary-care clinics in six academic medical centers from North Carolina, Florida, and Vermont were surveyed about a variety of topics including their preferences for religious/spiritual involvement in their own medical encounters. While two-thirds thought that their physician should be aware of their religious or spiritual orientation, only one-third wanted to be asked about this during a routine office visit. Not surprisingly, the more severe the medical condition, the more willing the patients were to consider a spiritual or religious interaction. Thus, 50 percent thought it would be appropriate in a near-death situation. However, only 19 percent believed it appropriate during a conventional office visit.

Importantly, these patients were asked questions that are not typically asked in other studies about their religious and spiritual preferences in medical care. They were asked whether they would want their doctor to discuss spiritual issues *even if it meant spending less time on their medical problems.* When asked in this way, the numbers of patients who wanted spiritual discussions as part of their medical care plummeted. Only 10 percent reported that they were willing to make this trade-off, while 78 percent were not. If other researchers asked the question in this way—making it clear that a trade-off was involved—the percentage of responses in favor of bringing spiritual and religious interactions into clinical medicine would be even lower than reported.

This handful of studies appears to be the basis for assertions about the enormous demand for physicians to address spiritual matters in clinical practice. Not only are there very few, but in most of the studies, only a minority of those surveyed reported that they were interested in religious or spiritual involvement in their medical care. And in the most representative of these reports, only 1 percent of the respondents reported that they would choose a physician from among the multiple people with whom they might discuss spiritual concerns. In fact, reading the original studies themselves instead of the secondary reports by advocates yields an entirely different picture about patient demand. In previous chapters we saw how misleading secondary sources have been in reporting accurately the data on associations between religion and health. They appear to be no more accurate when the issue is patient demand.

Thus, like most of the claims in the religion-and-health literature, the evidence that there is a clamor for bringing religious activities into clinical medicine is overstated. In most studies, fewer than half of the subjects expressed this interest, and the narrow limits of these studies suggest that generalization to all medical practice is unwarranted. To make matters more complicated, family practice physicians report lack of time (71 percent), inadequate training (59 percent), and difficulty identifying patients who want to discuss spiritual issues (56 percent) as significant barriers to raising these issues.

But let's assume for the moment that these surveys accurately reflect the desire among most patients to bring religion into medical practice, and ask another provocative question: Is a patient's request for more religious attention in medical practice enough of a reason for a physician to attempt to incorporate the two? Patients often ask for things that are unrealistic and/or that may not be in their best interests. Heart disease patients often express the desire to continue eating a high-fat diet when caloric restriction and a low-fat diet are called for. Diabetics want to continue to eat sugary foods when it is unwise for them to do so. Cancer patients may wish to discontinue chemotherapy before it is appropriate. Physicians often confront cases in which hospitalized patients request discharge against medical advice. In these cases, as in other clinical situations, the decision to accede to these wishes is complex and requires weighing the conflicting bioethical principles of beneficence (the responsibility to act to further the patient's good as the physician sees it) and autonomy (the patient's right to act independently in an informed manner). The mere fact that some patients may want physicians to engage in religious activities with them is not enough, per se, to justify it.

Dr. David Larson, who urged us to tear down the wall of separation between religion and medicine, commented that we should address religious and spiritual matters in clinical medicine because patient surveys indicate a desire for this. Like so many other statements in the field, this one is exaggerated and misleading. There is no evidence of an outpouring of desire on the part of the patient community for establishing closer links between religion and medicine. Even when there is an interest, it generally is expressed only by a minority of patients or applies only to very narrow circumstances, and it declines precipitately when patients are asked to choose between discussion of religious matters and medical ones. Like the claims that evidence supports associations between religion and health, the claims of high levels of patient demand for bringing religious practices into clinical medicine are simply wrong.

# 13

## TRIVIALIZING THE TRANSCENDENT:
## BE CAREFUL WHAT YOU WISH FOR

**We've now seen that efforts to bring religion and** spirituality into clinical medicine are justified by neither the evidence about the relationship between religion and health nor the data on patient demand. In addition, there are significant ethical problems that arise from efforts to do so. And, for several different reasons, it's not practical, either. But it is abundantly clear that attempts to link religion to health are widespread and increasing nonetheless. In this chapter, we'll consider the relationship between religion and health from a different perspective altogether: that efforts to use the methods of science to study religion demean, even trivialize, the religious experience. We'll consider this problem in three different ways:

1. By implementing the approach of scientific reductionism, the transcendent aspects of the religious experience are diminished if not lost altogether.
2. Satisfying the scientific demand for general consensus on the measurement of religious variables results in "dumbing down" religion by eliminating what is distinctive about different religious traditions.

3. Using the methods of science to establish the relative merits of different religious traditions reflects the "value-free" scientific materialism that many deplore.

Recall from the discussions about research methods covered earlier in the book that science depends completely upon the capacity to measure the phenomena it studies. If something can't be measured, it can't be studied scientifically. Sometimes this isn't difficult. If we're interested in the effect of a new drug on cholesterol levels, we can specify precisely the amount of the drug we give to subjects. Similarly, we can measure the impact of that drug on blood cholesterol with great accuracy. Measurement of the independent variable (the drug) and the dependent variable (blood cholesterol) is simple and unambiguous.

But many of the interesting questions we'd like to ask in biomedicine involve variables that are not so easy to measure. This certainly is the case for the scientific examination of religion and spirituality. To study them, we have to measure them—to somehow quantify them—and unfortunately, there are no simple blood counts or drug levels to help us. Our measurement procedures have the effect of reducing religion and spirituality to relatively crude indices. Thus, attendance at religious services has become the most widely used index of religiosity, not because it perfectly captures the experience of religious devotion but rather because it is easy to measure. We simply ask people to report how frequently they attend.

We've already addressed the problems inherent in getting people to report accurately on religious attendance when we interview them, because of their need to preserve a certain image in the face of the interviewer. We've also considered the fact that people attend religious services for a variety of reasons, many of which have nothing to do with religious devotion: they like the social contact, they have long-standing habits based in their family histories, they lack anything better to do on Saturday or Sunday morning, or they are interested in developing business contacts, to name only a few. And even if these other influences didn't exist, attendance would still represent only a single behavior that encompasses a tiny fraction of the whole of the religious or spiritual experience. In other words, the measurement requirements of science reduce religion and spirituality to something that does not represent them fully and as a result does violence to them. Here's another example that illustrates this point rather dramatically.

In a recent issue of the *American Journal of Psychiatry*, researchers from the Karolinska Institute in Stockholm demonstrated that there were significant relationships between activity of the serotonin system in the brain and spiritual and religious inclinations. Specifically, they found an inverse relationship between a measure of self-transcendence, a personality characteristic that covers religious behavior and attitudes, and the density of serotonin receptors in several brain regions. To translate: greater religious behavior and stronger religious experience were associated with fewer serotonin receptors located in several parts of the brain. Serotonin, a neurotransmitter, has long been the focus of researchers interested in personality and behavior. The Swedish researchers concluded that the serotonin system may be the biological basis of spiritual experiences, i.e., *religiosity and spirituality are the products of brain neurochemistry.*

To fully understand these findings, we need to delve a bit into some basic facts and findings from the field of neurochemistry. Neurotransmitters are chemical messengers that convey information from cell to cell in the brain and nervous system. Because these cells are separated from each other by small spaces called *synapses,* some mechanism is required to transfer information across the synapse, thus allowing that information to continue along its path. Neurotransmitters like serotonin, norepinephrine, and dopamine accomplish this objective.

Neurotransmitters typically are found in small pockets called *vesicles* in the end of a *neuron,* a nervous system cell. When a neuron is stimulated, the electrochemical message travels from one end of the cell to the other, causing these vesicles to move within the neuron to the end of the cell that borders on the synapse. The vesicle fuses with the cell membrane, releasing the neurotransmitter into the synapse. It crosses the synapse to the next cell, binding to *receptors* on the surface of the postsynaptic cell, where, depending upon the type of neurotransmitter, it either initiates an electrochemical impulse in this cell or acts to inhibit this impulse. That is, after the neurotransmitter binds to the receptor, it either causes the cell to fire or inhibits its firing.

The effect of the neurotransmitter depends substantially on its remaining in the synapse. One way to regulate its activity is to control how long it stays there. Two notable mechanisms influence this: enzymatic degradation and reuptake. If an enzyme degrades the transmitter, i.e., breaks it down, then it can no longer perform its transmission function of conveying information from one neuron to the next. The second mechanism, reuptake, involves returning the transmitter to the presynaptic cell. If the transmitter is no longer in the synapse, it is no longer biologically active. The activity of the neuron depends in part on the state of the receptors on the postsynaptic surface. The denser the collection of receptors—the more of them there are per square unit of cell surface—the greater the likelihood that the neurotransmitter will bind and cause the nerve cell to respond.

Serotonin is one of many neurotransmitters in the brain. Its activity has been implicated in many human activities and experiences, the most widely known of which is depression. According to current thinking in psychiatry, depression is the product of altered activity of the serotonin system. This could be the result of release of too little serotonin from the presynaptic vesicles. Or it could be that there are too few serotonin receptors on the postsynaptic cell. Or it could be that something is removing serotonin from the synapse too quickly. Regardless of which of these is operative, they all result in insufficient serotonin signaling, and insufficient serotonin signaling is what, current thinking holds, accounts for depression. Of course, this explanation is oversimplified, but it will do for our purposes.

The way to address this problem is to produce more serotonin in the synapse, and this is precisely what we think the most popular antidepressant drugs do. They are called selective serotonin reuptake inhibitors or SSRIs. What SSRIs do is block reuptake of serotonin. Ordinarily, the serotonin released into the synapse returns to the presynaptic vesicles through the process of reuptake. But SSRIs block this process, presumably resulting in more serotonin in the synapse. More serotonin in the synapse means more serotonin signaling, and according to theory, this has an antidepressant effect.

Now let's return to the Swedish study linking brain serotonin to religiosity and spirituality. Borg and colleagues found that in three regions of the brain, the raphe nucleus, the hippocampus, and the neocortex, density of the serotonin receptors on the postsynaptic cell was lower in subjects in whom religiosity was higher. One consequence of this is reduced serotonin signaling—fewer receptors means lower serotonin binding, and binding is related to the activity of the neuron. Imagine, by comparison, that there are one thousand people telephoning an office to send a message but there are only two people answering the phone in that office. Most of the messages won't get through. In precisely the same way, if there is lots of serotonin in the synapse but very few receptors to accept it, then the neural message won't get through. The findings are striking in another regard: they are highly similar to the profile of serotonin receptor function in patients with panic disorder. That is, both patients with high levels of religiosity and patients with panic disorder have the same pattern of reduced density of serotonin receptors in these regions of the brain.

Advocates of a connection between religion and health clamor for scientific studies to explore this association. The Borg paper clearly is one such study. Are the advocates satisfied with studies that link religious experience to brain neurochemistry in a way that makes it the neurochemical cousin of a psychiatric disorder? Is that all there is to it? Should we now consider the possibility that the passion of Jesus Christ was merely the product of serotonin activity in the brain? Would the course of religious history be different if Buddha had taken an SSRI?

Such suggestions seem blasphemous, but they derive directly from attempts to link religion and medicine by scientific investigation. Ironically, these attempts result in precisely the reductionist scientific materialism that religious conservatives and liberals alike deplore. The Swedish study is by no means the only one to pursue a reductionist strategy that results in trivializing religion. In recent years, a field called *neurotheology* has emerged. Using the techniques of neuroimaging, neurotheology aims to identify the biological basis for religious and spiritual experiences.

As you might expect, this combination of high-tech brain imaging and spirituality captured the attention of the media, and neurotheology landed on the cover of the May 7, 2001, issue of *Newsweek*. The article reported on the studies of neurologist Andrew Newberg and colleagues at the University of Pennsylvania, who used a technology called SPECT to identify regions of the brain that were activated during Buddhist meditation.

SPECT stands for single photon emission computed tomography. It is one of several brain-imaging techniques that are used to detect the activity of different regions of the brain. Like the more commonly used positron-emission tomography (PET), SPECT detects the presence of small amounts of radioactivity emitted from a radiopharmaceutical injected into a vein or artery. These radiopharmaceuticals are created to bind preferentially to areas of the body that are the most active. Depending on the circumstances, some parts of the brain are more active than others, and these more active areas will take up more of this radiopharmaceutical. SPECT brain imaging uses a gamma camera that acquires images as it moves around the head detecting areas of the brain that emit more or less gamma radiation. The amount of radiation they emit depends upon how much of the radiopharmaceutical they have taken up, which depends in turn on how active they are. The multiple images from the camera are assembled by a computer to create a three-dimensional picture of the brain that reflects the activity of different brain regions.

Dr. Newberg and his colleague Dr. Eugene d'Aquili reported, not surprisingly, that brain areas associated with concentration and attention, two hallmarks of meditation, showed increased activity compared to other regions. Regions of the brain associated with the sense of space and time showed reduced activity, consistent with the experience of the loss of the sense of self characteristic of meditation. These entirely unremarkable findings were similar to findings by the same authors in a study of Christian prayer. Newberg and d'Aquili ask us to consider whether these images of brain activity are a "photograph of God."

Based largely on these two small studies with a total of eleven subjects, Newberg and d'Aquili went on to write *Why God Won't Go Away*, a book that speculates broadly about these modest findings. The title of the book suggests that the authors will use their research in neuroimaging to reveal important existential truths about religious and spiritual experiences. Although *Why God Won't Go Away* is not organized in this way, Newberg and d'Aquili present three propositions:

1. Mystical religious experiences are based on the activity of the brain.
2. Because of this, these experiences are real.
3. "Neurology can reconcile the rift between science and religion, by showing them to be powerful but incomplete pathways to the same ultimate reality."

Let's examine each of these.


## MYSTICAL RELIGIOUS EXPERIENCES ARE BASED ON THE ACTIVITY OF THE BRAIN

Newberg and d'Aquili write that "the profound spiritual experiences described by saints and mystics of every religion, and in every period of time, can also be attributed to the brain's activity." The central thesis is that the ecstatic experiences and visions of religious mystics through-out history have neurological underpinnings. This, they believe, tells us that the brain is "wired" for religion and spirituality.

It is true, of course, that throughout history, religious mystics have had ecstatic experiences and visions. But ancient mystics are not the only ones who have these experiences. New Age spiritualist Dr. Doreen Virtue has written twenty books in which she describes having conversations with angels who provide her with advice on topics as distinct as healing and eating chocolate. Apparently, she converses with them all the time. David Berkowitz, the famous "Son of Sam" murderer in the late 1970s, heard voices from his dog Sam telling him to kill. The defendants at the Salem witchcraft trials of 1692 also reported out-of-body experiences and visions similar to those described by mystics. If Newberg and d'Aquili could have conducted brain-imaging studies of David Berkowitz or the "witches" of Salem, they also would have found increased activity in the same regions of the brain that light up during meditation and prayer. In fact, we know this already. Imaging studies of people with schizophrenia show that many of the same areas are activated during hallucinations.

Saints and mystics are not the only ones who experience ecstatic religious states. In the August 29–September 5, 2005, issue of *Newsweek* magazine, the cover story devoted to spirituality in America reported on the experience of Ron Cox, who was raised in the Southern Baptist tradition but left it in his teens. He then tried Hinduism and Buddhism, but neither resonated with him. "But one summer night recently, guided by the voice of God to a Pentecostal revival in full-throated swing, he was transfixed by the sight of worshipers so moved by the Holy Spirit that they were jumping, shouting and falling to the floor in a faint. Soon he, too, was experiencing the ecstasy of the Holy Spirit. It seemed to lift him right out of his body." Clearly, experiences of religious ecstasy are not restricted to true mystics.

Here's the important thing: there is nothing at all remarkable about reporting that ecstatic religious experiences are associated with a neurological substrate. Lighting up regions of the brain in a PET or SPECT scan image doesn't give them any special significance. *All* human conscious activity, religious or otherwise, has an underlying counterpart in brain activity. The act of reading this book and the hallucinations of schizophrenics are associated with underlying brain activity—not necessarily the *same* brain activity but brain activity nonetheless. Using advanced neuroimaging techniques to demonstrate that there are changes in the activity of the prefrontal cortex or inferior parietal lobes during religious experience sheds no particular light on the transcendent aspects of religion. It merely reflects increased metabolism of certain brain regions. But the effort to identify the biological substrates of religious experience tells us a great deal about the reductionist nature of the neurotheology enterprise (we'll come back to this in a few moments).

## BECAUSE THESE EXPERIENCES ARE ASSOCIATED WITH BRAIN ACTIVITY, THEY ARE REAL

Newberg and d'Aquili contend that because these mystical religious experiences are attributable to underlying brain activity, they are real. Consider, for example, their account of Margareta Ebner, a fourteenth-century German nun. After quoting a passage from her journal in which she writes that she was "grasped by an inner divine power of God," they ask, "Could it be that Sister Margareta really was visited by the mystical presences of Jesus. . . . Or was she, as most modern, rationalistic thinkers would insist, the victim of some emotional or psychological imbalance?"

Fortunately, Newberg and d'Aquili answer this question for us. "Our own scientific research, however, suggests that genuine mystical encounters like Sister Margareta's are not necessarily the result of emotional distress or neurotic delusion or any pathological state at all." Because mystical experiences are associated with a neurological substrate, Newberg and d'Aquili believe, they are not the result of neurotic delusion or emotional distress. If they are not delusions, the authors imply, they must be real. But this manner of distinguishing a real experience from a delusion doesn't help us at all, because we saw above that *all* human experience depends in some way upon brain activity. Every experience is real if we define "real" merely as corresponding to a biological substrate. No experience can be a delusion if this is our definition.

This causes a significant problem. Is there any reason not to apply the same logic to a twenty-first-century New Age spiritual guru, or a person whose mental illness produces hallucinations, that Newberg and d'Aquili apply to a fourteenth-century nun? The fact that Sister Margareta's experience could be shown to be associated with changes in underlying brain activity does not make her experience true or false, delusional or real. The auditory hallucinations of schizophrenia also are associated with underlying brain activity similar, no doubt, to the brain activity in Sister Margareta.

Having a biological substrate, therefore, does not make an experience real. Our modern understanding of dreams makes this abundantly clear. We call them *dreams* precisely because we don't believe they are real, but with contemporary neuroimaging techniques, we can examine the underlying brain activity associated with them. Researchers from the NIH have done precisely this. So the fact that an experience is associated with the activity of the brain tells us nothing at all about whether something is real or not.

## NEUROLOGY CAN RECONCILE THE RIFT BETWEEN SCIENCE AND RELIGION

Finally, Newberg and d'Aquili contend that their research will allow us to reconcile the gap between science and religion. This reconciliation, it appears, is based on the previous "insight" that religious and spiritual experiences that have their basis in brain activity must be real. Following this logic, science, which also is based on the neurological activity of the brain, also must be real. But at the same time, they write, science is "a type of mythology, a collection of explanatory stories that resolve the mysteries of existence." Like all other human experiences, science is filtered through the human brain and therefore has no greater claim to objectivity than any other experience. Science, like religion, is real but based entirely on subjectivity.

Newberg and d'Aquili are by no means the only people to have considered that science is the product of the human brain and therefore has no particular claim to the truth. The postmodernist critique of science, as a human activity influenced like all other human activities by social forces, especially power relationships, essentially makes the same claim. This postmodernist position is associated with another characteristic, relativism, that Newberg and d'Aquili's position directly implies. If what makes our experience valid is its neurological basis, then my insights have no greater claim to reality than yours. All truths are relative.

The problem with this account, and with Newberg and d'Aquili's claims that they thus have reconciled the difference between science and religion, is the identification of the validity of an experience with its neurological substrate. The paranoid's claim that he is receiving messages from the CIA via a transmitter implanted in a dental filling is no less valid than the claims Newberg and d'Aquili make about science and religion. Since they all are based on an underlying neurological reality, they are equally valid.

In taking this approach, Newberg and d'Aquili obscure rather than reconcile the essential difference between science and religion in a way that doesn't satisfy either. Even though both are associated with neurological substrates, they employ different approaches to the truth. Their neurological origins are irrelevant. Conventional wisdom says that religious truths are based on faith that does not require the empirical validation provided by SPECT scans or any of the other methods of science. For the devout, the validity of Sister Margareta's vision does not depend upon identifying the activity of the region of the brain associated with it. Her vision is accepted without this "validation."

Validation in science, on the other hand, depends completely on systematic empirical observation. Scientific insights have corresponding neurological substrates, and these are "filtered" through the brain, like all human experience, but this is entirely irrelevant. Facts in science are based on agreement that they represent the best account of observations collected in an acceptably systematic and unbiased fashion. Applying the methods of neuroimaging does not reconcile religion and science. Rather, it misunderstands the fundamental distinction between them.

There is another problem with the "reconciliation" proposed by Newberg and d'Aquili. By suggesting that both religion and science are the products of brain activity and therefore ultimately subjective, Newberg and d'Aquili strip from religion one of its central characteristics: the capacity to speak of universal truths. To be sure, different religions have different universal truths, but this does not obscure the fact that appealing to the universal is a central feature of religion. Implying that the "truth" is established by neurological validation is precisely the position of moral relativism that religion opposes.

The failure to distinguish these essential differences between science and religion, along with the reduction of mystical experiences to underlying brain neurochemistry, is yet another example of the trivializing of the transcendent. The suggestion that we can take a photograph of God using the technology of neuroimaging would be funny if it wasn't so grandiose. This approach should be deeply disturbing to theologians, and more generally to people of faith, regardless of their religious orientation.

Thus, neurotheology offers us nothing at all. It cannot, as Newberg and d'Aquili assert, tell us anything about the distinction between science and religion. It cannot tell us whether mystical religious visions are real in the conventional sense or not. It most definitely cannot tell us anything at all about the existence of God.

This kind of reductionism—the view that all human experience can be reduced to the function of biological activity—may be satisfying to scientists, but it is anathema to theologians. Researchers

Marguerite Lederberg and George Fitchette recognized this problem in an interesting article with the provocative title "Can You Measure a Sunbeam with a Ruler?" In it, they explore the scientific problems with attempts to reduce the experience of religion to the measurable quantities of science. The point of their title is to reiterate a long-standing concern in science: the difficulty of quantifying human experience. By attempting to measure a sunbeam and in so doing reduce it to that which can be quantified by a ruler, we lose the character of the sunbeam itself. While such measurement may be possible, it cannot capture the essence of the sunbeam and in fact may distort it.

Trying to quantify religious experience by counting the number of times a person reports attending church, the most commonly used index of religious involvement, is like trying to measure a sunbeam with a ruler: it may be possible, but the essential character of the experience is lost in the process. It is like trying to quantify the aesthetic experience of listening to a Beethoven symphony by counting the number of times a listener smiles. No doubt we could conduct brain-imaging studies to demonstrate differences in the activity of cerebral structures while listening to the Ninth Symphony and to white noise. Would that tell us anything about the aesthetic experience? Would it mean that this experience is explained by the activity of that specific brain region? Is that all there is to it? Is the majesty of listening to Beethoven, viewing the Grand Canyon, or appreciating the vastness of the universe merely the product of increased activity of certain regions in the brain? And could we reproduce these experiences simply by administering the right medication or electrical stimulation?

As productive as this strategy of reductionism has been and as promising as it continues to be for science, we ought to question seriously what insights it yields in the study of religion. As we have emphasized throughout this book, religion and science are independent approaches to knowledge, and neither can be reduced to the other. Religion and science are fundamentally different, with the former relying on faith as a source of wisdom and the latter demanding evidence.

Religious truths generally are considered to be enduring and not subject to change. Scientific truths, on the other hand, are completely dependent on evidence, and as new evidence emerges, scientific truths change accordingly.

For these reasons, attempts to understand religious experience by scientific means can *never* be satisfying to religion. They can satisfy only science.

## DUMBING DOWN RELIGION

Using the methods of science to study religion and spirituality is troublesome in another respect. It relates not so much to biological reductionism as to the scientific requirement of objectifiable measurement standards. As a strategy, this works well for science. It does not work very well for religion. By seeking a common denominator in measurement, religion is "dumbed down," stripped of its most significant content.

This concern finds a parallel in the debate about church-state relationships in the U.S. In *Sleeping with Extra-Terrestrials,* Wendy Kaminer writes that "routine references to God, in the Pledge of Allegiance or on our currency, are constitutional precisely because, in the words of the late Supreme Court justice William Brennan, 'they have lost through rote repetition any significant religious content.'" That is, references to religion, to be acceptable to the religiously diverse population of the U.S., must be stripped of so much content that all meaning is eliminated.

Progress is made in medicine when previously disparate definitions of a condition are resolved in favor of a common one. We approve of, rather than condemn, the fact that we all can agree on what constitutes hypertension or hyperlipidemia, even if ultimately definition is arbitrary. But there is nothing particularly transcendent about levels of blood pressure or cholesterol. We don't object to efforts to develop a universally accepted standard. The situation is different with religion.

Molly Ivins has provided a wonderful example of how this problem affects religion. "By the time you get the Catholics, Jews, Episcopalians, Methodists, Muslims, atheists, agnostics, Church of Christers, Buddhists, Sikhs, New Agers and the County Line Salt of the Earth Church of the Predestinarian Faith to sign off on one prayer, it begins: 'To Whom It May Concern, If There Is a Whom.'" Although she wrote this comment about school prayer, it applies equally well to attempts to study religion scientifically. By the time we get around to establishing measures of religiosity that satisfy *everyone,* we have dumbed down the religious experience so much that it has become meaningless. It reminds me of the saying made famous during the Vietnam War: "In order to save the village, we had to destroy it."

This simplification made possible by the measurement requirements of science permits us to lump indices of religiosity with other important medical variables. Medicine has made great strides over the centuries, and as a result of these advances, physicians can now prescribe medications to control heart disease and cure infections. They can also recommend behaviors (e.g., eating a low-fat diet, getting regular exercise, not smoking) that have a significant impact on our health. Assuming that there was solid evidence of an association between religious activities and beneficial health outcomes, should medicine treat religious activities in the same way? Should physicians recommend attending church because it might promote health in the same way that regular exercise does? Is church attendance like getting regular exercise or consuming a low-fat diet?

Are the meaning and value of church attendance related solely to improving health? One does not need to be deeply religious, or even religious at all, to recognize that the behavior of attending religious services can have much greater significance than merely as an instrumental means to health improvement. In fact, we assume that attending religious services has a *transcendental* meaning, derived from a tradition of worship that relates religious acts to a divine presence. This is not true of consuming a low-fat diet. Attending religious services is valued, independent of any health effects it might produce. To suggest or even imply that doctors should treat religious activities in the same way they treat health behaviors profoundly demeans the former.

## CONTRASTING THE RELATIVE MERITS OF DIFFERENT RELIGIONS

Using the methods of science to examine religion has another seemingly unintended consequence: it has led to attempts to establish the relative merits of different religious traditions by scientific means. After all, if you can determine scientifically whether frequency of attendance or frequency of prayer is associated with health outcomes, then shouldn't we begin to test whether the type of service makes a difference? If we are truly interested in collecting information relevant to health outcomes, then we should want to know whether it is better for our health to attend a Catholic Mass or a Quaker meeting. Are Orthodox Jewish services better for our health than Reform services? Is there a health advantage to praying five times a day, as Muslims do, as opposed to the three times of Orthodox Jews? Why is it acceptable to determine that more frequent attendance at religious services is better for your health than less frequent attendance, but it is not acceptable to determine that Christian services are better for your health than attending Jewish or Muslim services?

Of course, the advocates of bringing religion into clinical medicine object to this approach. They report that no one would consider this, because it is so offensive. But some *have* considered it: "Science has demonstrated in three separate studies the efficacy of Christian prayer in medical studies. There is no 'scientific' (non-spiritual) explanation for the *cause* of the medical effects demonstrated in these studies. The only logical, but not testable, explanation is that God exists and answers the prayers of Christians. No other religion has succeeded in scientifically demonstrating that prayer to their God has any efficacy in healing." There is no ambiguity about this statement. It makes it clear that the author believes that the effect of prayer to the Christian God has been validated scientifically. No other religion, he writes, can make that claim. The implication is straightforward: Christianity is superior to all other religions. The dangers of this view are obvious.

Unfortunately, the author of this Web site article is not alone in clamoring for studies to document the relative merits of different religious denominations. In the *The Lancet,* an editorial accompanying the report of the entirely negative MANTRA II trial of distant intercessory prayer asked, "Could a more restricted denominational approach have influenced the outcome?" Somewhat obliquely, *The Lancet* editorially was asking whether the study might have detected an effect of distant prayer if it had examined denominational prayer, e.g., Christian or Jewish, instead of the heterogeneous mixture examined in MANTRA II. Asking this question is tantamount to endorsing efforts to compare the effects of the prayers of different religious denominations.

Dr. Harold Koenig and his colleagues also endorse this position, at least in the case of mental health. "Studies are needed to determine whether different religious beliefs have similar effects on the course and outcome of mental disorders. Does the impact of religion depend on whether one is Jewish, Christian, Muslim, Buddhist, Hindu, atheist, or a New Age believer? . . . Prospective studies are needed."

Dr. Herbert Benson is more cautious. He has said that it doesn't make any difference which religious rituals you practice, only that you practice some, to gain the health benefits. "My review of the research reveals that regardless of how traditional one's practice of religious beliefs, whenever faith is present . . . health can be improved." But this statement puts him in a peculiar position. First of all, he has no evidence for it. No scientific evidence comparing the health benefits of different religious traditions has been reported in the medical literature. For those who insist that they rely on evidence when promoting the health benefits of religious experience, this is an odd departure. But even this statement by Benson doesn't actually argue against the idea of comparing scientifically the effects of rituals of different religious denominations or traditions.

Most researchers in the field of religion and health do not address this matter. My guess is that if they were asked, they would oppose contrasting the health benefits of different religious denominations. But why should they object? Presumably, the objection to studying the different health effects of Christianity, Judaism, and Islam, for example, is that it would be offensive if we discovered that one religion was superior to the other two. The offense lies in the implication that those who practice the medically less beneficial religions would be better off converting to the medically more beneficial one.

Such a recommendation would be seen as out of bounds by most people. But why should it be? Attending services at an Orthodox synagogue or a Catholic church is a religious behavior that we can measure, just like attending services more or less frequently. Why is recommending conversion from one religious denomination to another for hypothetical health benefits more offensive than recommending that people who attend services only once per month attend more frequently because the latter, some believe, is better for their health, or recommending that people increase the amount of time spent praying?

Dr. Koenig appears to have no reluctance to make recommendations about increasing one's religious activities. As we saw in Chapter 10, he offers precisely this advice. To those who already are religious, he advises going to services more frequently. To the same people, he advises awakening thirty minutes earlier each day and spending that extra time in prayer. Koenig is not alone in his willingness to recommend changes in deeply personal religious activities in the service of providing health benefits. Dr. David Larson felt the same way. He wrote a paper entitled "Clinical Religious Research, How to Enhance Risk of Disease: Don't Go to Church."

It's not clear from the literature how many others in the field feel this way. Few are as bold as Koenig or Larson. Nevertheless, the problem remains. In each of these cases, scientific evidence is being used to encourage a change in a deeply personal religious practice. It doesn't matter that the evidence is poor in quality. What's important is the effort to encourage the change, whether that change relates to converting from one religion to another or converting from one religious practice like attendance at services or prayer to another.

We are on dangerous ground here, and the danger lies once again in a critical distinction between science and religion. It is a distinction that proponents of the religion-health connection obliterate, whether they intend to or not. Science permits us, in principle, to answer these questions. Without a doubt, we could conduct a study contrasting the health effects of Christianity, Judaism, and Islam, for example. It could be done in precisely the same way that researchers have examined the effects of higher versus lower frequency of attendance at religious services or greater or lower frequency of private prayer or reading the Bible or listening to religious radio programming. From the *scientific* perspective, there is no fundamental difference between using religious denomination or religious attendance as the predictor variable. Of course, such a study would be subject to the same problems of observational studies that we've already addressed. But in this matter, these problems are irrelevant.

Although science allows us to conduct such a study, ethics and religion ought to tell us how ridiculous such a comparison would be. In today's world (and in the past as well), we have ample evidence of religious strife. This should not diminish the value that religion has for many people, but no one can dismiss the fact that religious factionalism has been responsible for conflict at the societal and familial level for thousands of years. Even if we could, hypothetically, demonstrate that Protestant prayer is better for one's health than Catholic prayer, why would we ever want to do so?


It undoubtedly is true that we can submit religious ritual and experiences to scientific study to determine if they are associated with beneficial health outcomes. But to do so runs the risk of trivializing the religious experience, making it no different from other medical recommendations made by physicians. If attending religious services becomes no different than consuming a low-fat diet or getting regular exercise, a great deal will have been lost. Bringing religion into the world of the scientist must by definition reduce religion to measurable indices that strip it of the sense of transcendence that distinguishes it from other aspects of our lives. Doing this dumbs religion down, making it so bland and universally acceptable that it has lost all of its meaning.

Ironically, this reductionism is precisely the problem that many in the religious community have railed against. Steven Goldberg, author of *Seduced by Science,* wrote, "When prayer is innocuous, it is no rival to the materialistic view of the world." Bringing religion into the "laboratory" of the scientist cannot help but contribute to the inevitable comparisons of the "scientifically established" virtues of one religion, or one type of religious practice, over others. Breaking down the wall between religion and health, as Larson and Matthews urge us to do, is fraught with perils they have not considered. In a world riven with religious factionalism and strife, it's hard to think of a worse idea.

# PART FOUR

Conclusions

# 14

## RELIGION AND MEDICINE: HOPE OR HYPE?

**Religion and science share a complex history and a** complex present as well. In various places around the world and at various times, medical and spiritual care were dispensed by the same person. In other eras, passionate—even violent—conflicts characterized the relationship between religion on the one hand and medicine and science on the other. Where do things stand at the beginning of the twenty-first century?

In the introduction, three questions about efforts to closely link religion and medicine were posed:

1. Do these efforts to link religion and health represent good science?
2. Do they represent good medicine?
3. Do they represent good religion?

As we have seen, the answer to all three question is no.

Despite the very poor quality of the studies that claim to show relationships between religious devotion and better health; despite the serious ethical problems that arise when physicians attempt to bring religion into clinical care; despite the fact that if busy practicing physicians engage in religious inquiries with patients, they won't have enough time to address the better-documented risk factors like smoking, exercise, diet, and stress; despite the fact that attempting to study religion using the methods of science trivializes the transcendent aspects of religion; despite all these reasons why it's a *bad idea* to link religious practices and clinical medicine, *there is no dispute that for a great many people, religion brings comfort in times of difficulty,* whether the difficulty is related to illness or something else.

Is this a contradiction? Not at all. Identifying the many problems with attempts to link religion and medicine doesn't diminish for a moment the capacity of religion to provide comfort to the suffering. Throughout this book, we have returned repeatedly to the fact that religion and science represent different approaches to knowledge, wisdom, and truth, each with its own operating principles. This does not make one superior to the other. But it does make them different. Science and religion exist as largely independent domains.

Recognizing the effort to bring religion into clinical medicine as bad science, bad medicine, and bad religion is not a critique of religion at all. In fact, it's an effort to protect religion against the trivialization of being simply another part of the scientific enterprise.

Consider the comment of astrophysicist Neil deGrasse Tyson, the director of the Hayden Planetarium in New York City and one of the nation's leading planetary scientists: "The methods of science have little or nothing to contribute to ethics, inspiration, morals, beauty, love, hate, or aesthetics. These are vital elements of civilized life and are central to the concerns of nearly every religion." Tyson makes it clear that there are essential domains of human existence that are beyond the means of science to address. For religion, on the other hand, these concerns are central. Attempting to use religion in clinical medicine as just another medical tool, like an antibiotic or a stent, relegates it to a subordinate position relative to science. Attempting to demonstrate scientifically the "value" of attending religious services or personal prayer abandons the very distinction between science and religion that speaks to these essential human characteristics.

Those who attempt to bring religion into the laboratory of science, who attempt to take a "photograph of God," who claim that religious involvement will lower your blood pressure, who tell us that prayer will influence medical outcomes of patients at a great distance, who use the privileged authority inherent in the role of the doctor to manipulate the religiosity of vulnerable and fearful patients, forget the advantage of religion over science in these characteristics that Tyson describes. They appear to believe that religion has no strengths of its own and instead needs to use the methods of science to establish its validity. In these efforts, they demean rather than defend religion.

People have successfully used religious ritual in times of trouble for thousands of years, and they will continue to do so for many thousand more. The key for us is to recognize that they do it on their own, or with their family, friends, and clergy. There is no doubt that in this way, religious ritual provides comfort and hope to many.

The problem arises when physicians attempt to become involved. That's when questions of evidence, ethics, and efficiency arise. If physicians make claims to patients about the benefits of religious activities, then the patients can feel manipulated or even coerced into engaging in religious behaviors that are not their own, to please their doctors. The case of the Colorado surgeon "requesting" that patients pray with him just before surgery makes it clear how manipulative this can be. In a country that values religious freedom as much as anything else, coercive religious practices are unacceptable. And physicians risk transgressing other ethical boundaries when they link religious practices with health outcomes. They invade the privacy of patients, and they can actually cause harm, as we saw in Chapter 10.

All of us, sooner or later, will succumb to illness and death. Some will die prematurely. Others will live longer than expected. For many, illness will raise important religious and spiritual concerns, providing comfort to some and anxiety to others. No one disputes the significance of these concerns, whether they arise in times of illness or at other times of distress. But recognizing that religious and spiritual concerns arise in times of illness doesn't mean that doctors should take these concerns on as part of their responsibility. As we have already seen, doctors lack the time, the training, and the experience to engage in spiritual interactions with patients.

When patients raise religious concerns about their health, doctors should do what they routinely do when they lack relevant expertise: they should refer the patients to the appropriate specialist. When a patient has complicated heart disease, we expect a doctor to refer him or her to a cardiologist. When a patient has a complex neurological problem, we expect that patient will be referred to a neurologist. Why would we expect anything less for a patient with religious and spiritual concerns? Fortunately, just as there are medical specialists who treat complex heart and neurological diseases, there are specialists with experience in religious and spiritual matters. We call them clergy, and doctors should refer patients with religious concerns to them no less readily than they refer patients with complex cardiac arrhythmias to cardiologists.

The title of this concluding chapter—"Religion and Medicine: Hope or Hype?"—suggests that there is an answer to this question. Is it hope that religious devotion is associated with health benefits? Or is it hype? In fact, the field of religion and health is characterized by both.

In his interesting book, *The Anatomy of Hope,* Dr. Jerome Groopman, an oncologist at Harvard, wrote that physicians should always encourage hope in their patients, even when there is little reason to be optimistic. We can *hope* for the best even if we don't expect it. That's a subtle but important distinction. We don't know if there are any medical benefits of hope. But we certainly know that the quality of patients' lives is better with hope than without it.

In the eighteenth century, Goethe wrote, "In all things it is better to hope than to despair." For many, religion is one source of hope for the best when illness makes our lives cruel, frightening, and unpredictable. But hoping for something is not the same as expecting it to happen.

# NOTES

## Chapter 1: Introduction

4 "What can I do . . .": D. A. Matthews, M. E. McCullough, D. B. Larson, H. G. Koenig, J. P. Swyers, and M. G. Milano, "Religious Commitment and Health Status," *Archives of Family Medicine* 7 (1998): 123.

5 Over half of U.S. medical schools: J. S. Levin, D. B. Larson, and C. M. Puchalski, "Religion and Spirituality in Medicine: Research and Education," *JAMA* 278 (1997): 792–93.

5 Harvard physician Herbert Benson: H. Benson, *Timeless Healing* (New York: Fireside, 1996).

5 Physicians David Larson and Dale Matthews: D. A. Matthews and D. B. Larson, "Faith and Medicine: Reconciling the Twin Traditions of Healing," *Mind/Body Medicine* 2 (1997): 3–6.

5 "the medicine of the future . . .": H. Sides, "The Calibration of Belief," *New York Times Magazine,* December 7, 1997, 85.

6 Harold Koenig and colleagues: H. G. Koenig, M. E. McCullough, and D. B. Larson, *Handbook of Religion and Health* (New York: Oxford University Press, 2001).

6 An earlier claim: D. A. Matthews and C. Clark, *The Faith Factor* (New York: Viking, 1998).

7 A 1996 poll: T. McNichol, "The New Faith in Medicine," *USA Today,* April 7, 1996.

7 Biomedical researcher David Eisenberg: D. M. Eisenberg, R. C. Kessler, C. Foster, F. E. Norlock, D. R. Calkins, and T. L. Delbanco, "Unconventional Medicine in the United States: Prevalence, Costs, and Patterns of Use," *New England Journal of Medicine* 328 (1993): 246–52.

8 New York Academy of Sciences: P. R. Gross, N. Levitt, and M. W. Lewis, eds., *The Flight from Science and Reason* (New York: New York Academy of Sciences, 1997).

9 University of Kentucky psychiatrist: N. Scheurich, "Reconsidering Spirituality and Medicine," *Academic Medicine* 78 (4) (2003): 360.

9 In a thoughtful critique: J. T. Chibnall, J. M. Jeral, and M. A. Cerullo, "Experiments on Distant Intercessory Prayer: God, Science, and the Lesson of Massah," *Archives of Internal Medicine* 161 (21) (2001): 2529–36.

9 In his compelling book: S. Goldberg, *Seduced by Science: How American Religion Has Lost Its Way* (New York: New York University Press, 1999).

9 The Reverend Joe Baroody: J. Baroody, "Faith Versus Death: The Problem with Medicine's Faith Factor Theology," *Journal of the South Carolina Medical Association* 97 (8) (2001): 347–52.

10 Chaplains Thomas O'Connor and Elizabeth Meakes: T. S. J. O'Connor, "Religion and Health Research: Critique of Critique Not Well Balanced," *Journal of Pastoral Care and Counseling* 57 (1) (2003): 85–86.

10 Writing from the perspective: H. Heffernan, "Religion and Health Research: Interpretation Sends Wrong Message Regarding Need for Hospital Chaplains in Health Care Institutions," *Journal of Pastoral Care and Counseling* 57 (1) (2003): 79–81.

## Chapter 3: From *Sputnik* to Angels

27 As a recent op-ed: D. Beynton, "'Intelligent Design' Deja Vu," *Washington Post*, December 17, 2005.

30 As Paul Dickson: P. Dickson, *"Sputnik": The Shock of the Century* (New York: Walker, 2001).

31 "You suddenly made us . . .": Quoted in ibid., 223.

32 The cover of the November: "Knowledge Is Power," *Time*, November 18, 1957.

36 "Scientists take themselves . . .": D. C. Dennett, "Postmodernism and Truth," in D. O. Dahlstrom, ed., *The Proceedings of the Twentieth World Congress of Philosophy* (Bowling Green, OH: 2000), 99–100.

39 Jacob Cohen: J. Cohen, *Statistical Power Analysis for the Behavioral Sciences* (Hillsdale, NJ: Erlbaum, 1988).

46 According to the review: G. Pion and M. W. Lipsey, "Public Attitudes Toward Science and Technology: What Have the Surveys Told Us?" *Public Opinion Quarterly* 45 (1981): 303–316.

46 "We might conclude . . .": Ibid., 313.

46 Other survey data: A. Lawler, "Support for Science Stays Strong," *Science* 272 (5266) (1996): 1256.

47 Surveys commissioned by: National Science Foundation, *Science and Engineering Indicators 2004*, http://www.nsf.gov/statistics/seind04/c7/c7s2.htm#note27.

47 More than 70 percent: National Science Foundation, *Science and Engineering Indicators* (Arlington, VA: National Science Foundation, 2000).

48 "All we know . . .": Wendy Kaminer, *Sleeping with Extra-Terrestrials* (New York: Vintage Books, 1999), 100.

48 "The therapeutic culture . . .": Ibid., 176.

49 "Flights from reason . . .": L. Gilkey, "The Flight from Reason: The Religious Right," in P. R. Gross, N. Levitt, and M. W. Lewis, eds., *The Flight from Science and Reason* (New York: New York Academy of Sciences, 1997).

49 A June 8, 2001, Gallup poll: F. Newport and M. Strausberg, "Americans' Belief in Psychic and Paranormal Phenomena Is Up over Last Decade," http://poll.gallup.com/content/default.aspx?ci=4483&pg=1.

49 A February 2002 CBS News poll: "Poll: Most Believe in Psychic Phenomena," CBS

News, April 28, 2002, http://www.cbsnews.com/stories/2002/04/29/opinion/polls/main507515.shtml.

49  Similarly, a Harris poll: H. Taylor, "The Religious and Other Beliefs of Americans, 2003," February 26, 2003, http://www.harrisinteractive.com/harris_poll/index.asp?PID=359.

49  Data from a June 16: D. Moore, "Three in Four Americans Believe in Paranormal," http://poll.gallup.com/content/default.aspx?ci=16915&pg=1.

## Chapter 4: Why Now?

55  *Mary Duffy was lying:* B. Carey, "In the Hospital, a Degrading Shift from Person to Patient," *New York Times,* August 16, 2005.

56  According to a recent survey: Kaiser Family Foundation, *National Survey on Consumers' Experiences with Patient Safety and Quality Information* (Menlo Park, CA: Kaiser Family Foundation, 2004).

58  More recently, José Pagán: J. A. Pagán and M. V. Pauly, "Access to Conventional Medical Care and the Use of Complementary and Alternative Medicine," *Health Affairs (Millwood)* 24 (1) (2005): 255–62.

66  On August 23, 1998: G. P. Posner, "Has Science Proven the Divine Health Benefits of Religion?" *USA Today,* August 23, 1998.

67  "I was scheduled . . .": "Answered prayers," *U.S. News & World Report,* December 20, 2004, 57.

69  According to economist Robert Fogel: R. W. Fogel, *The Fourth Great Awakening and the Future of Egalitarianism* (Chicago: University of Chicago Press, 2000).

## Chapter 5: Are There Really So Many Studies on Religion and Health?

73  "the vast majority . . .": W. L. Larimore, M. Parker, and M. Crowther, "Should Clinicians Incorporate Positive Spirituality into Their Practices? What Does the Evidence Say?" *Annals of Behavioral Medicine* 24 (2002): 69–73.

73  Dr. Harold Koenig: H. G. Koenig, "Religion, Spirituality, and Medicine: Application to Clinical Practice," *JAMA* 284 (2000): 1708.

74  Mayo Clinic physician Paul Mueller: P. S. Mueller, D. J. Plevak, and T. A. Rummans, "Religious Involvement, Spirituality, and Medicine: Implications for Clinical Practice," *Mayo Clinic Proceedings* 76 (12) (2001): 1226.

74  Dr. Dale Matthews: Matthews et al., "Religious Commitment and Health Status," *Archives of Family Medicine* 7 (1998): 118–24.

76  Thus, for example, according to: R. T. Walden, L. E. Schaefer, F. R. Lemon, A. Sunshine, and E. L. Wynder, "Effect of Environment on the Serum Cholesterol-Triglyceride Distribution Among Seventh-Day Adventists," *American Journal of Medicine* 36 (1964): 269–76.

77  For example, Dr. Jeff Levin: J. S. Levin, J. S. Lyons, and D. B. Larson, "Prayer and Health During Pregnancy: Findings from the Galveston Low Birthweight Survey," *Southern Medical Journal* 86 (1993): 1022–27.

77  In another study: M. A. McColl, J. Bickenbach, J. Johnston, S. Nishihama, M. Schumaker, K. Smith et al., "Spiritual Issues Associated with Traumatic-Onset Disability," *Disability & Rehabilitation* 22 (12) (2000): 555–64.

78 "Occupational Stress . . .": E. H. Friedman and H. K. Hellerstein, "Occupational Stress, Law School Hierarchy, and Coronary Artery Diseases in Cleveland Attorneys," *Psychosomatic Medicine* 30 (1968): 72–86.

78 Similarly, Dr. George Comstock: G. W. Comstock, "Fatal Arteriosclerotic Heart Disease, Water Hardness at Home, and Socioeconomic Characteristics," *American Journal of Epidemiology* 94 (1971): 1–10.

## Chapter 6: How Good Is the Evidence?

82 For example, a recent study: M. S. Mahonen, P. McElduff, A. J. Dobson, K. A. Kuulasmaa, and A. E. Evans, "Current Smoking and the Risk of Non-fatal Myocardial Infarction in the WHO MONICA Project Populations," *Tobacco Control* 13 (3) (2004): 244–50.

85 Ironically, a recent report: R. B. Turner, R. Bauer, K. Woelkart, T. C. Hulsey, and J. D. Gangemi, "An Evaluation of Echinacea Angustifolia in Experimental Rhinovirus Infections," *New England Journal of Medicine* 353 (4) (2005): 341–48.

86 "the prayers of the world . . .": J. Krakauer, *Under the Banner of Heaven: A Story of Violent Faith* (New York: Random House, 2003), 44.

86 "I don't think . . .": D. E. Murphy, "Utah Girl, 15, Is Found Alive 9 Months After Kidnapping," *New York Times,* March 13, 2003.

86 Extrapolating from 1999 data: D. Finkelhor, H. Hammer, and A. J. Sedlack, "Nonfamily Abducted Children: National Estimates and Characteristics," U.S. Department of Justice, report #196467, 1–16.

86 Martha, we read, expected: Matthews and Clark, *Faith Factor,* 70–71.

87 The National Cancer Institute's: National Cancer Institute, "Salivary Gland Cancer (PDQ®): Treatment" (2003).

87 a paper published in 1991: C. C. Wang and M. Goodman, "Photon Irradiation of Unresectable Carcinomas of the Salivary Glands," *International Journal of Radiation Oncology Biology & Physics* 21 (3) (1991): 569–76.

88 mesothelioma, a rare: K. H. Antman, "Current Concepts: Malignant Mesothelioma," *New England Journal of Medicine* 303 (4) (1980): 200–202.

91 Crisco is a . . . : S. J. Gould, *The Mismeasure of Man* (New York: Norton, 1981), 200.

92 "we know what happened . . .": Ibid., 233.

94 But when the trials: V. Beral, E. Banks, and G. Reeves, "Evidence from Randomised Trials on the Long-Term Effects of Hormone Replacement Therapy, *Lancet* 360 (9337) (2002): 942–44.

94 An influential review: W. C. Willett, "Vitamin A and Lung Cancer," *Nutrition Reviews* 48 (5) (1990): 201–11.

94 Regrettably, the results: "Alpha-Tocopherol Beta Carotene Cancer Prevention Study Group: The Effect of Vitamin E and Beta Carotene on the Incidence of Lung Cancer and Other Cancers in Male Smokers," *New England Journal of Medicine* 330 (15) (1994): 1029–35.

96 For instance, it is: See N. J. Christenfeld, R. P. Sloan, D. Carroll, and S. Greenland, "Risk Factors, Confounding, and the Illusion of Statistical Control," *Psychosomatic Medicine* 66 (6) (2004): 868–75:

97 In a recent study, 85 percent: M. Kuri, Y. Hayashi, K. Kagawa, K. Takada, T. Kamibayashi, and T. Mashimo, "Evaluation of Diagonal Earlobe Crease as a Marker

of Coronary Artery Disease: The Use of This Sign in Pre-operative Assessment,"
*Anaesthesia* 56 (12) (2001): 1160–62.

97 "voodoo science": R. L. Park, *Voodoo Science* (New York: Oxford University Press, 2000).

98 But according to journalist Po Bronson: P. Bronson, "A Prayer Before Dying," *Wired,* December 2002.

100 Consider an article by Hughes Helm: H. M. Helm, J. C. Hays, E. P. Flint, H. G. Koenig, and D. G. Blazer, "Does Private Religion Activity Prolong Survival? A Six-Year Follow-up Study of 3,851 Older Adults," *Journal of Gerontology* 55A (2000): M400–M406.

## Chapter 7: Is There Really a Health Advantage to the Religiously Active?

109 According to Robert Park: R. L. Park, "The Seven Warning Signs of Bogus Science," *Chronicle of Higher Education,* January 31, 2003.

109 On June 15, 2005: L. K. Altman, "Studies Rebut Earlier Report on Pledges of Virginity," *New York Times,* June 15, 2005, A21.

110 "a treatment discipline . . .": M. W. Krucoff, S. W. Crater, C. L. Green, A. C. Maas, J. E. Seskevich, J. D. Lane et al., "Integrative Noetic Therapies as Adjuncts to Percutaneous Intervention During Unstable Coronary Syndromes: Monitoring and Actualization of Noetic Training (MANTRA) Feasibility Pilot," *American Heart Journal* 142 (5) (2001): 761.

111 "gently touched the patient . . .": Ibid., appendix.

113 "the combination of the bedside . . .": E. Agnvall, "You Use That Stuff, Too?" *Washington Post,* June 29, 2004.

117 In 2003, Lynda Powell: L. H. Powell, L. Shahabi, and C. E. Thoresen, "Religion and Spirituality: Linkages to Physical Health," *American Psychologist* 58 (1) (2003): 36–52.

118 Carney and others: R. M. Carney, K. E. Freedland, and D. S. Sheps, "Depression Is a Risk Factor for Mortality in Coronary Heart Disease," *Psychosomatic Medicine* 66 (6) (2004): 799–801.

120 "at least 18 prospective studies . . .": Mueller et al., "Religious Involvement," 1226.

121 Drs. Jeffrey Levin and Harold Vanderpool: J. S. Levin and H. Y. Vanderpool, "Is Religion Therapeutically Significant for Hypertension?" *Social Science and Medicine* 29 (1989): 69–78.

121 "the characteristics and functions . . .": Ibid., 64.

122 Yechiel Friedlander and Jeremy Kark: Y. Friedlander and J. D. Kark, "Familial Aggregation of Blood Pressure in a Jewish Population Sample in Jerusalem Among Ethnic and Religious Groupings," *Social Biology* 31 (1–2) (1984): 75–90.

123 "The most important discoveries . . .": L. Dossey, "Prayer and Medical Science: A Commentary on the Prayer Study by Harris et al. and a Response to Critics," *Archives of Internal Medicine* 160 (12) (2000): 1736.

124 For example, physicians David Larson: Matthews and Larson, "Faith and Medicine."

124 "the medicine of the future . . .": Sides, "Calibration of Belief," 85.

124 "Do religious beliefs . . .": Koenig et al., *Handbook,* 5.

124 "I believe the practice . . .": W. L. Larimore, "Providing Basic Spiritual Care for

Patients: Should It Be the Exclusive Domain of Pastoral Professionals?" *American Family Physician* 63 (1) (2001): 40.

124 "'To exclude God . . .'": Ibid.

124 "This is no routine paper . . .": B. Carey, "Can Prayers Heal? Critics Say Studies Go Past Science's Reach," *New York Times,* October 10, 2004.

125 "In this era . . .": D. A. Matthews, D. B. Larson, and C. Barry, *The Faith Factor: An Annotated Bibliography of Clinical Research on Spiritual Subjects* (Rockville, Md.: National Institute of Healthcare Research, 1993), introduction (unpaginated).

127 One review examining: F. Luskin, "Review of the Effect of Spiritual and Religious Factors on Mortality and Morbidity with a Focus on Cardiovascular and Pulmonary Disease," *Journal of Cardiopulmonary Rehabilitation* 20 (1) (2000): 8–15.

127 The other is the voluminous: Koenig et al., *Handbook.*

127 "evidence continues to mount . . .": Luskin, "Review of the Effect," 8.

127 "of the 16 studies . . .": Koenig et al., *Handbook,* 263.

128 Koenig's study of attendance: H. G. Koenig, L. K. George, J. C. Hays, D. B. Larson, H. J. Cohen, and D. G. Blazer, "The Relationship Between Religious Activities and Blood Pressure in Older Adults," *International Journal of Psychiatry in Medicine* 28 (1998): 189–213.

128 One found that subjects: T. W. Graham, B. H. Kaplan, J. Cornoni-Huntley, S. A. James, C. Becker, C. G. Hames et al., "Frequency of Church Attendance and Blood Pressure Elevation," *Journal of Behavioral Medicine* 1 (1978): 37–43.

128 The other study: D. B. Larson, H. G. Koenig, B. H. Kaplan, R. S. Greenberg, E. Logue, and H. A. Tyroler, "The Impact of Religion on Men's Blood Pressure," *Journal of Religion and Health* 28 (1989): 265–78.

128 One, a study of patients: E. McSherry, M. Ciulla, S. Salisbury, and D. Tsuang, "Spiritual Resources in Older Hospitalized Men," *Social Compass* 35 (1987): 515–37.

129 The problem is: T. E. Oxman, D. H. Freeman, and E. D. Manheimer, "Lack of Social Participation or Religious Strength and Comfort as Risk Factors for Death After Cardiac Surgery in the Elderly," *Psychosomatic Medicine* 57 (1995): 5–15.

129 (all of which . . . ): E. L. Idler and S. V. Kasl, "Religion Among Disabled and Nondisabled Persons II: Attendance at Religious Services as a Predictor of the Course of Disability," *Journal of Gerontology* 52B (1997): S306–S316.

129 One suggested health benefits: R. C. Harris, M. A. Dew, A. Lee, M. Amaya, L. Buches, D. Reetz et al., "The Role of Religion in Heart-Transplant Recipients' Long-Term Health and Well-Being," *Journal of Religion and Health* 34 (1995): 17–32.

129 The final paper: T. L. Saudia, M. R. Kinney, K. C. Brown, and L. Young-Ward, "Health Locus of Control and Helpfulness of Prayer," *Heart Lung* 20 (1) (1991): 60–65.

130 Emilia Bagiella's and my: R. P. Sloan and E. Bagiella, "Claims About Religious Involvement and Health Outcomes," *Annals of Behavioral Medicine* 24 (1) (2002): 14–21.

131 After reviewing these thirty-four: Ibid.

131 a paper by Jane Leserman: J. Leserman, E. M. Stuart, M. E. Mamish, and H. Benson, "The Efficacy of the Relaxation Response in Preparing for Cardiac Surgery," *Behavioral Medicine* 15 (3) (1989): 111–17.

131 Sudsuang et al.: R. Sudsuang, V. Chentanez, and K. Veluvan, "Effect of Buddhist Meditation on Serum Cortisol and Total Protein Levels, Blood Pressure, Pulse Rate, Lung Volume and Reaction Time," *Physiology and Behavior* 50 (3) (1991): 543–48.

132 "walking about 1 km . . .": Ibid., 544.

132 Michael Cooper and Maurice Aygen: M. J. Cooper and M. M. Aygen, "A Relaxation Technique in the Management of Hypercholesterolemia," *Journal of Human Stress* 5 (4) (1979): 24–27.

133 Another study, by Barry Blackwell: B. Blackwell, S. Bloomfield, P. Gartside, A. Robinson, I. Hanenson, H. Magenheim et al., "Transcendental Meditation in Hypertension: Individual Response Patterns," *Lancet* 1 (7953) (1976): 223–26.

133 Wenneberg et al.: S. R. Wenneberg, R. H. Schneider, K. G. Walton, C. R. Maclean, D. K. Levitsky, J. W. Salerno et al., "A Controlled Study of the Effects of the Transcendental Meditation Program on Cardiovascular Reactivity and Ambulatory Blood Pressure," *International Journal of Neuroscience* 89 (1–2) (1997): 15–28.

133 a study by Miller: R. N. Miller, "Study on the Effectiveness of Remote Mental Healing," *Medical Hypotheses* 8 (5) (1982): 481–90.

134 "a gifted individual . . .": Ibid., 482.

134 "contact the inner mind . . .": Ibid., 484.

134 "who had the highest . . .": Ibid., 486.

135 One of my favorite examples: S. K. Kumanyika and J. B. Charleston, "Lose Weight and Win: A Church-Based Weight Loss Program for Blood Pressure Control Among Black Women," *Patient Education and Counseling* 19 (1) (1992): 19–32.

135 "techniques commonly used": Ibid., 22.

136 Hixson et al.: K. A. Hixson, H. W. Gruchow, and D. W. Morgan, "The Relation Between Religiosity, Selected Health Behaviors, and Blood Pressure Among Adult Females," *Preventive Medicine* 27 (4) (1998): 545–52.

136 Koenig himself: H. G. Koenig, D. O. Moberg, and J. N. Kvale, "Religious Activities and Attitudes of Older Adults in a Geriatric Assessment Clinic," *Journal of the American Geriatrics Society* 36 (4) (1988): 362–74.

136 The third study: K. L. Lapane, T. M. Lasater, C. Allan, and R. A. Carleton, "Religion and Cardiovascular Disease Risk," *Journal of Religion and Health* 36 (1997): 155–63.

136 "overall, we found . . .": Ibid., 162.

138 The table below lists: Powell et al., "Religion and Spirituality."

## Chapter 8: Attendance at Services and Mortality

148 Kirk Hadaway and colleagues: D. K. Hadaway, P. L. Marler, and M. Chaves, "What the Polls Don't Show: A Closer Look at U.S. Church Attendance," *American Sociological Review* 58 (1993): 741–52.

149 Other researchers of attendance: M. Chaves and J. C. Cavendish, "More Evidence on U.S. Catholic Church Attendance," *Journal for the Scientific Study of Religion* 33 (1994): 376–81.

149 Stanley Presser: S. Presser and L. Stinson, "Data Collection Mode and Social Desirability Bias in Self-Reported Religious Attendance," *American Sociological Review* 63 (1998): 137–45.

149 "I would like to ask . . .": Ibid., 139.

149 According to Hadaway: C. K. Hadaway, P. L. Marler, and M. Chaves, "Over-reporting Church Attendance in America: Evidence That Demands the Same Verdict," *American Sociological Review* 63 (1) (1998): 127.

150 But they may operate: R. Torurangeau and T. Smith, "Asking Sensitive Questions: The Impact of Data Collection Mode, Question Format, and Question Context," *Public Opinion Quarterly* 60 (1996): 275–304.

150 Indeed, when questions: Presser and Stinson, "Data Collection."

## Chapter 9: Why Long-Distance Healing Doesn't Have a Prayer

158 The entirely negative results: H. Benson, J. A. Dusek, J. B. Sherwood et al., "Study of the Therapeutic Effects of Intercessory Prayer (STEP) in Cardiac Bypass Patients: A Multicenter Randomized Trial of Uncertainty and Certainty of Receiving Intercessory Prayer," *American Heart Journal* 151 (2006): 934–42.

159 The best-known study: R. C. Byrd, "Positive Therapeutic Effects of Intercessory Prayer in a Coronary Care Unit Population," *Southern Medical Journal* 81 (1988): 826–29.

161 Dr. William Harris and colleagues: W. S. Harris, M. Gowda, J. W. Kolb, C. P. Strychacz, J. L. Vacek, P. G. Jones et al., "A Randomized, Controlled Trial of the Effects of Remote, Intercessory Prayer on Outcomes in Patients Admitted to the Coronary Care Unit," *Archives of Internal Medicine* 159 (1999): 2273–78.

162 "This result suggests . . .": Ibid., 2274.

162 My colleague Emilia Bagiella: R. P. Sloan and E. Bagiella, "Data Without a Prayer," *Archives of Internal Medicine* 160 (12) (2000): 1870; discussion 1877–78.

167 According to a news release: T. Koepke, "Prayer, Noetic Studies Feasible; Results Indicate Benefit to Heart Patients," DukeMedNews, October 31, 2001, http://www.dukemednews.org/news/article.php?id=5056#top.

168 Theological critics: C. B. Cohen, S. E. Wheeler, D. A. Scott, B. S. Edwards, P. Lusk, and the Anglican Working Group in "Bioethics: Prayer as Therapy," *Hastings Center Report* 30 (2000): 40–47.

168 (STEP study): Benson et al., "Study."

169 But in IP studies: Cohen et al., "Prayer."

170 We have no idea: Chibnall et al., "Experiments on Distant Intercessory Prayer."

170 Jeffrey Dusek and colleagues: J. A. Dusek, J. B. Sherwood, R. Friedman, P. Myers, C. F. Bethea, S. Levitsky, P. C. Hill, M. K. Jain, S. L. Kopecky, P. S. Mueller, P. Lam, H. Benson, P. L. Hibberd, "Study of the Therapeutic Effects of Intercessory Prayer (STEP): Study Design and Research Methods," *American Heart Journal* 143 (2002): 577–84.

171 Why, this criticism goes: Cohen et al., "Prayer."

171 As Stephen Black put it: S. L. Black, "The Finger of God," *British Medical Journal* 324 (2002): 1037.

171 Larry Dossey: L. Dossey, "Prayer and Medical Science: A Commentary on the Prayer Study by Harris et al. and a Response to Critics." *Archives of Internal Medicine* 160 (12) (2000): 1735–37.

172 "We need not wait . . .": Dossey, "Prayer and Medical Science," 1737.

172 "an effective adjunct . . .": Harris et al., "Randomized, Controlled Trial," 2274.

172 Byrd, Harris, and STEP: Byrd, "Positive Therapeutic Effects"; Harris et al., "Randomized, Controlled Trial"; Dusek et al., "Study of the Therapeutic Effects."
172 Because of the lack: Chibnall et al., "Experiments on Distant Intercessory Prayer."
172 as Dr. Joseph Chibnall recommends: Ibid.
173 "While it is true . . .": Dossey, "Prayer and Medical Science," 1736.
173 "there is considerable evidence . . .": Ibid., 1735.

## Chapter 10: Ethical Problems

184 Even in the twenty-first century: Gould, *Mismeasure*; J. Groopman, "Your Cancer Isn't Your Fault," *New York Times*, April 21, 2000.
187 the now-discredited eugenics: Gould, *Mismeasure*.
189 McCaffrey and colleagues: A. M. McCaffrey, D. M. Eisenberg, A. T. R. Legedza, R. B. Davis, and R. S. Phillips, "Prayer for Health Concerns: Results of a National Survey on Prevalence and Patterns of Use," *Archives of Internal Medicine* 164 (8) (2004): 858–62.
190 She recommends the following: C. M. Puchalski, "Spirituality and Health: The Art of Compassionate Medicine," *Hospital Physician*, March 2001, 30–36.
190 Dr. Harold Koenig recommends: H. G. Koenig, "An 83-Year-Old Woman with Chronic Illness and Strong Religious Beliefs," *JAMA* 288 (4) (2002): 490.
191 Indeed, as Dr. Neil Scheurich: Scheurich, "Reconsidering Spirituality."
192 marital status and health: S. Ebrahim, G. Wannamethee, A. McCallum, M. Walker, and A. Shaper, "Marital Status, Change in Marital Status, and Mortality in Middle Aged British Men," *American Journal of Epidemiology* 142 (1995): 834–42.
192 Socioeconomic status also: N. E. Adler, T. Boyce, M. A. Chesney, S. Cohen, S. Folkman, R. L. Kahn et al., "Socioeconomic Status and Health: The Challenge of the Gradient," *American Psychologist* 49 (1994): 15–24.
192 early rather than late childbearing: M. Lambe, M. Thorn, P. Sparen, R. Bergstrom, and H. O. Adami, "Malignant Melanoma: Reduced Risk Associated with Early Childbearing and Multiparity," *Melanoma Research* 6 (1996): 147–53; J. M. Ramon, J. M. Escriba, I. Casas, J. Benet, C. Iglesias, L. Gavalda et al., "Age at First Full-Term Pregnancy, Lactation and Parity and Risk of Breast Cancer: A Case-Control Study in Spain," *European Journal of Epidemiology* 12 (1996): 449–53.
193 "What can I do . . .": Matthews et al., "Religious Commitment," 123.
196 *The Healing Power of Faith*: H. G. Koenig, *The Healing Power of Faith* (New York: Simon & Schuster, 1999), 280–81, 277–78.
197 *The Saline Solution*: W. L. Larimore and W. C. Peel, *The Saline Solution: Sharing Christ in a Busy Practice* (Bristol, TN: Paul Tournier Institute, 2000).
198 "If we could have . . .": Ibid., 115.
198 *I went to a new*: Ibid., 33.
199 *To a patient facing*: Ibid., 84.
199 "faith stories": Ibid., 88.
199 *When we were pregnant*: Ibid.
199 *It may surprise you*: Ibid., 96.
199 "Remember that you're . . .": Ibid., 85.
200 Doctors receive the following: Ibid., 119, 97, 88.
200 "Raising faith flags . . .": Ibid., 118.
201 "over ten years . . .": Ibid., 108.

201 "You know from . . .": Ibid., 94.

202 Today, the primary focus: T. L. Beauchamp and J. F. Childress, *Principles of Biomedical Ethics* (New York: Oxford University Press, 2001).

204 A recent study about prostate: H. Cohen and N. Britten, "Who Decides About Prostate Cancer Treatment? A Qualitative Study," *Family Practice* 20 (6) (2003): 724–29.

205 "religion flourishes . . .": Quoted in G. Wills, *Under God* (New York: Simon & Schuster, 1990), 379.

205 "churches freed . . .": Ibid., 25.

## Chapter 11: Is It Practical to Bring Religion into Medicine?

207 "must seek to understand . . .": Association of American Medical Colleges, *Report I: Objectives for Medical School Education: Guidelines for Medical Schools* (Washington, DC: Association of American Medical Colleges, 1998), 50.

208 Koenig provides an illustration: Koenig, "An 83-Year-Old."

208 "Keep it up!": Ibid., 491.

209 "groups like the Posse Comitatus": N. Rosenblum, *Membership and Morals* (Princeton, NJ: Princeton University Press, 1998).

210 "by inquiring about . . .": Puchalski, "Spirituality and Health," 35.

210 "Physicians need, however . . .": A. B. Astrow, C. M. Puchalski, and D. P. Sulmasy, "Religion, Spirituality, and Health Care: Social, Ethical, and Practical Considerations," *American Journal of Medicine* 110 (4) (2001): 284.

212 What qualifies them: G. Anandarajah and E. Hight, "Spirituality and Medical Practice: Using the HOPE Questions as a Practical Tool for Spiritual Assessment," *American Family Physician* 63 (1) (2001): 81–89.

212 "positive spirituality": W. L. Larimore, M. Parker, and M. Crowther, "Should Clinicians Incorporate Positive Spirituality into Their Practices? What Does the Evidence Say?" *Annals of Behavioral Medicine* 24 (1) (2002): 71.

213 "honesty, self-control . . .": Ibid.

213 "that separate people . . .": Ibid.

214 "a social movement . . .": P. Skrabanek, "Preventive Medicine and Morality," *Lancet* 1 (8473) (1986): 143.

214 "There are many . . .": Ibid., 144.

215 Susan Sontag: S. Sontag, *Illness as Metaphor* (New York: Farrar, Straus & Giroux, 1978).

215 They require an expansion: Anandarajah and Hight, "Spirituality and Medical Practice."

216 Focusing only on: R. Lawrence, "The Witches' Brew of Spirituality and Medicine," *Annals of Behavioral Medicine* 24 (2002): 74–76.

217 Breast Cancer: D. A. Berry, K. A. Cronin, S. K. Plevritis, D. G. Fryback, L. Clarke, M. Zelen et al., "Effect of Screening and Adjuvant Therapy on Mortality from Breast Cancer," *New England Journal of Medicine* 353 (17) (2005): 1784–92.

218 According to a recently published: K. S. H. Yarnall, K. I. Pollak, T. Ostbye, K. M. Krause, and J. L. Michener, "Primary Care: Is There Enough Time for Prevention?" *American Journal of Public Health* 93 (4) (2003): 635–41.

218 For example, another recent study: M. T. Ruffin, D. W. Gorenflo, and B. Woodman, "Predictors of Screening for Breast, Cervical, Colorectal, and Prostatic

Cancer Among Community-Based Primary Care Practices," *Journal of the American Board of Family Practice* 13 (1) (2000): 1–10.

219 Another recent study examined: T. Ostbye, K. S. H. Yarnall, K. M. Krause, K. I. Pollak, M. Gradison, and J. L. Michener, "Is There Time for Management of Patients with Chronic Diseases in Primary Care?" *Annals of Family Medicine* 3 (3) (2005): 209–14.

220 only 10 percent of them: C. D. MacLean, B. Susi, N. Phifer, L. Schultz, D. Bynum, M. Franco et al., "Patient Preference for Physician Discussion and Practice of Spirituality: Results from a Multicenter Patient Survey," *Journal of General Internal Medicine* 18 (1) (2003): 38–43.

220 In the *Handbook*: Koenig et al., *Handbook*.

226 According to religious historian Diana Eck: D. Eck, *A New Religious America* (New York: HarperCollins, 2001).

227 Thomas O'Connor and Elizabeth Meakes: O'Connor, "Religion and Health Research."

## Chapter 12: Is There Really a Demand for Bringing Religion into Medicine?

232 "In 1994, 96 percent . . .": Koenig et al., *Handbook*, 4.

232 "According to a 1990 . . .": Benson, *Timeless Healing*, 173.

232 "national surveys repeatedly show . . .": J. Levin, *God, Faith, and Health* (New York: John Wiley & Sons, 2001), 20.

232 "polls indicate that . . .": Koenig, *Healing Power*, 25.

232 According to the World Values Survey: N. Knox, "Religion Takes a Back Seat in Western Europe," *USA Today*, August 11, 2005.

234 religious attendance dropped: Presser and Stinson, "Data Collection Mode."

235 For example, researchers Dana King and Bruce Bushwick: D. E. King and B. Bushwick, "Beliefs and Attitudes of Hospital Patients About Faith, Healing, and Prayer," *Journal of Family Practice* 39 (1994): 349–52.

235 Drs. Todd Maugans and Willcom Wadland: T. Maugans and W. C. Wadland, "Religion and Family Medicine: A Survey of Physicians and Patients," *Journal of Family Medicine* 32 (1991): 210–13.

235 Timothy Daaleman and Donald Nease: T. Daaleman and D. Nease, "Patients' Attitudes Regarding Physician Inquiry into Spiritual and Religious Beliefs," *Journal of Family Practice* 39 (1994): 564–68.

235 "we should address . . .": David Larson, quoted in L. Gunderson, "Faith and Healing," *Annals of Internal Medicine* 132 (2000): 170.

236 Ehman et al. reported: J. W. Ehman, B. B. Ott, T. H. Sort, R. C. Ciampa, and J. Hansen-Flaschen, "Do Patients Want Physicians to Inquire About Their Spiritual or Religious Beliefs If They Become Gravely Ill?" *Archives of Internal Medicine* 159 (1999): 1803–6.

237 Mansfield and colleagues reported: C. J. Mansfield, J. Mitchell, and D. E. King, "The Doctor as God's Mechanic? Belief in the Southeastern United States," *Social Science & Medicine* 54 (2002): 399–409.

237 456 patients from primary-care: MacLean et al., "Patient Preference."

238 To make matters more complicated: M. R. Ellis, D. C. Vinson, B. Ewigman, "Addressing Spiritual Concerns of Patients: Family Physicians' Attitudes and Practices," *Journal of Family Practice* 48 (1999): 105–9.

239  In these cases: T. L. Beauchamp, "The Four-Principle Approach," in N. J. Lindemann and N. H. Lindemann, eds., *Meaning and Medicine: A Reader in the
Philosophy of Health Care* (New York: Routledge, 1999). 147–55.

## Chapter 13: Trivializing the Transcendent

243  researchers from the Karolinska: J. Borg, B. Andree, H. Soderstrom, and
L. Farde, "The Serotonin System and Spiritual Experiences," *American Journal of
Psychiatry* 160 (11) (2003): 1965–69.
245  Borg and colleagues found: Ibid.
245  The findings are striking: A. Neumeister, E. Bain, A. C. Nugent, R. E. Carson,
O. Bonne, D. A. Luckenbaugh et al., "Reduced Serotonin Type 1A Receptor
Binding in Panic Disorder," *Journal of Neuroscience* 24 (3) (2004): 589–91.
247  brain areas associated with: A. Newberg, A. Alavi, M. Baime, M. Pourdehnad,
J. Santanna, and E. d'Aquili, "The Measurement of Regional Cerebral Blood
Flow During the Complex Cognitive Task of Meditation: A Preliminary SPECT
Study," *Psychiatry Research* 106 (2) (2001): 113–22.
247  a study of Christian prayer: A. Newberg, M. Pourdehnad, A. Alavi, and E. G.
d'Aquili, "Cerebral Blood Flow During Meditative Prayer: Preliminary Findings
and Methodological Issues," *Perceptual and Motor Skills* 97 (2) (2003): 625–30.
247  three propositions: A. Newberg and E. d'Aquili, *Why God Won't Go Away* (New
York: Ballantine Books, 2001), 168–69.
247  "the profound spiritual experiences . . .": Ibid., 10.
248  The defendants at the Salem: G. Weissmann, "Sucking with Vampires": The Medicine of Unreason," in P. R. Gross, N. Levitt, and M. W. Lewis, eds., *The Flight
from Science and Reason* (New York: New York Academy of Sciences, 1996).
248  Imaging studies of people: B. R. Lennox, S. B. Park, I. Medley, P. G. Morris, and
P. B. Jones, "The Functional Anatomy of Auditory Hallucinations in Schizophrenia," *Psychiatry Research* 100 (1) (2000): 13–20.
248  "But one summer night . . .": J. Adler, "In Search of the Spiritual," *Newsweek*,
September 5, 2005, 46–64.
249  "grasped by an inner . . .": Newberg and d'Aquili, *Why God Won't Go Away*, 98.
249  "Could it be . . .": Ibid., 98–99.
249  "Our own scientific research . . .": Ibid., 100.
250  Researchers from the NIH: A. R. Braun, T. J. Balkin, N. J. Wesenten, R. E.
Carson, M. Varga, P. Baldwin et al., "Regional Cerebral Blood Flow Throughout
the Sleep-Wake Cycle: An H2(15)O PET Study," *Brain* 120 (pt. 7) (1997):
1173–97.
251  "a type of mythology . . .": Newberg and D'Aquili, *Why God Won't Go Away*, 170.
253  "Can You Measure . . .": M. S. Lederberg and G. Fitchett, "Can You Measure a
Sunbeam with a Ruler?" *Psychooncology* 8 (5) (1999): 375–77.
254  "routine references to God . . .": W. Kaminer, *Sleeping with Extra-Terrestrials*
(New York: Vintage Books, 1999), 54.
255  "By the time you get . . .": M. Ivins, *Prayer in Schools, Economic Stimulus, and
Other Nonsense* (Columbus, OH: Free Press, 2001).
256  "Science has demonstrated . . .": R. Deem, "Scientific Evidence for Answered
Prayer and the Existence of God," 2005, http://www.godandscience.org/apologetics/
prayer.html.

257 "Could a more restricted . . .": Anonymous, "Mantra II: Measuring the Unmeasurable?" *Lancet* 366 (9481) (2005): 178.

257 "Studies are needed . . .": Koenig et al., *Handbook,* 468.

257 "My review of the research . . .": Benson, *Timeless Healing,* 173.

258 "Clinical Religious Research . . .": S. S. Larson and D. B. Larson, "Clinical Religious Research, How to Enhance Risk of Disease: Don't Go to Church," *Christian Medical & Dental Society Journal* 23 (3) (1992): 14–19.

260 "When prayer is innocuous . . .": Goldberg, *Seduced by Science,* 91.

## Chapter 14: Religion and Medicine: Hope or Hype?

264 "The methods of science . . .": N. D. Tyson, "Holy Wars: An Astrophysicist Ponders the God Question," *Natural History* 2001 (1999), 80–82.

# INDEX

Christian Medical and Dental Association, 5–6, 197
Christian medicine, 201–2
Christianity
    American, 226
    early, 11
    health benefits of, proposed study, 258–59
    and history of medicine, 20–22
    and suffering, as essential, 20
    superior effectiveness of prayers of, claimed, 256–57
Church, the, authority of, 22, 83
church and state issue, 68–69, 195, 254
circulatory system, 24–25
clergy
    spiritual matters to be referred to, 266
    training of, 226–28
clinical services, recommended standard treatment protocols, 216–19
clinical trials, 94–95
Cohen, Alan, 50, 51
Cohen, Jacob, 39
coin toss experiments, 101–4
colds, echinacea and prevention of, 84–85
Cold War, 28–33
    and interest in science education, 11, 31–33
Columbia University, 42
complementary and alternative medicine (CAM), 58, 84, 86, 113
Comstock, Dr. George, 78, 81–83, 93
    study of church attendance and mortality, 81–83, 93, 95, 100, 120, 144
confounders, 92–95, 144–47
    statistical control of, 145–46
consciousness, claim to operate at a distance, 173–74
construct validity, 151–52, 163–64
control group, 37–39, 143
Cooper, Michael, 132
Copernican theory, 23, 83
Copernicus, 23
coronary artery disease
    sudden remission of, 67
    surgical treatment of, 75
coronary bypass surgery, 128

coronary care units (CCUs)
    intercessory prayer for patients of, studies, 159–64
    outcomes of, 159–64
"creation science," 35–36
cross-sectional studies, 138
cystic fibrosis, 54

Daaleman, Timothy, 235
d'Aquili, Dr. Eugene, 247–52
Darwinism, challenge to, 9, 176
data dredging, 121–22
Dawkins, Richard, 8
death
    defined as a health outcome, 115
    universality of, 265–66
Dennett, Daniel, 36
denominations, religious
    differences in efficacy of prayers, suggested study of, 168
    differences in health characteristics, 76, 130, 182
    predominant in a region, and increased attendance at church, 146–47
    studying the relative merits of, proposal, 256–59
depression
    and heart disease, 43, 118
    serotonin and, 244–45
diagnostic cardiac catheterization, 110
diagnostic tests
    insensitive administering of, 58
    over-ordering of, 57
Diana, Princess, 186
Dickson, Paul, 30
disease. See illness
dissection, history of, 22–23
distant healing, 157
    of AIDS, 98–99
    of high blood pressure, 133–34
    mechanism of, proposed, 171–74, 176
distant intercessory prayer. See intercessory prayer
divine intervention, 171
doctors. See physicians
"do no harm," 183
Dossey, Dr. Larry, 123, 171–72, 173
double-blind studies, 41–42
dreams, 250

George Washington Institute on
    Spirituality and Health (GWISH), 5
George Washington University Medical
    School, 5
Germans, 90
glioblastoma, study of, 4
God
    belief in, 7, 232
    "putting Him to the test," caution
        against, 14, 171
    taking a photograph of, 252
gods, as cause of illness, 17, 18, 20
God's will, illness as, 188, 211
Goethe, J. W. von, 267
Goldberg, Steven, 9, 260
Gould, Stephen Jay, 8, 88, 92, 152
"Great Awakenings," 68–70
Greeks, ancient, 11
    medicine of, 18–19, 215
    physicians of, in ancient Rome, 20
Green, Chad, 188–89
Groopman, Dr. Jerome, 266
Gruber, Jonathan, 146–47

Haddaway, Kirk, 148
Harris, Dr. William, 161–64, 172, 176
Harris Poll
    on belief in God, 233
    on paranormal phenomena, 49
Harvard Medical School, 4–5
Harvey, William, 19, 24–25
hate groups, and benefits to health from
    membership, conceivably, 209–10
healing, miraculous, 21
health
    attendance at church and, 78, 93, 95,
        99–100
    hate groups and, 209–10
    marriage and, 182
    private prayer and, 100
    religious involvement and, 77, 100,
        127–40, 189
    smoking and, 143–44, 153
    social assimilation and, 122
    socioeconomic status and, 192
    sports and, 191
health characteristics, denominational
    differences in, 76, 130, 182, 258–59
health insurance, 56, 99

health maintenance organizations
    (HMOs), 56
health outcomes
    death as one, 115
    life factors associated with, religion
        as one of many, 191–93
    weighting of, 162–64
heart disease
    depression and, 43, 118
    earlobe crease and, 97
    process of, 133
heart rate variability, 165
heart transplants, religious involvement
    and, 129
Heatter, Gabriel, 31
Heffernan, Henry, S.J., 10
Helms, Hughes, 100
herbal medicine, ancient, 15, 18
herbs, health claims for, 84
Heritage Foundation, 109
Hindu tradition, 132
Hippocrates, 18–19
Hippocratic oath, 183
history, medical
    doctors taking, 193
    See also spiritual history
Hixson, Karen, 136
"holistic," 49
hope, 266–67
hormone replacement therapy (HRT),
    health outcomes of, 94
hospitals
    early Christian, 21
    patient abuse in, 55–56
Hover, Margot, 192
Hummer, Robert, 141–42
humors, four, 19
Hungarians, 90
hypotheses, testing of, 35

illness
    basic questions people ask about, 15
    causes of, primitive beliefs about, 15,
        17, 18, 20
    as God's will, 188, 211
    Greek study of, 18–19
    moral responsibility for, belief in,
        17–18, 181, 184–87, 215
    prayer instead of medical care for, 189

imagery techniques, and cardiac
    procedures, 110
imaging of brain, 246–52
immigration policy, U.S., 1920s, 90–92,
    187
impact factor (of journals), 116–18
informed consent, 201–2
Institute for Scientific Information (ISI),
    116–17
insurance companies, 57
intelligence
    ethnicity and, 90–92
    IQ and, 152
    native and acquired, 90
intelligence testing
    and expected "blooming" of
        schoolchildren, 40–41
    and immigration policy, 90–92, 187
    and true intelligence, 152
intelligent design movement, 8–9,
    35–36, 176
Intelligent Design Network, 176
intercessory prayer (IP), 4, 98–99, 157–77
    and cardiac treatment, 111
    claims for, 123
    mechanism of, proposed, 171, 176
    negative results of studies of, 158
    studies of, 61, 159–71, 176–77
*International Journal of Psychiatry in
    Medicine (IJPM)*, 119
Internet, effect on journalism, 67
inter-rater reliability, 163–64
interview methods
    inaccuracy of, 142, 147–50, 233
    participants' answers in, 147
IQ, and intelligence, 152
Islam, health benefits of, proposed study,
    258–59
Italians, 90
Ivins, Molly, 255

Jefferson, Thomas, 205
Jesuits, 204
Jews
    American, 226
    health studies of, 76
    intelligence of, purported, 90
Johns Hopkins University, 81
    Department of Epidemiology, 81

Johnson, Lyndon, 30
John Templeton Foundation, 60–64, 168
Jones, Judge John, 36
journalism
    "pack," 66–67
    subjectivity in, 66
    uncritical, sensational, 66–68
*Journal of Cardiopulmonary
    Rehabilitation*, 127
*Journal of the American Medical
    Association (JAMA)*, 117
journals, medical
    impact factor of, 116–18
    peer-reviewed, 108
    relative quality of, 116–19
Judaism, ancient, religion-medicine
    practice in, 17–18
Judaism, modern, health benefits of,
    proposed study, 258–59
junk science, 97
just-world hypothesis, 185–87, 215

Kaminer, Wendy, 11
    *Sleeping with Extra-Terrestrials*,
        47–48, 254
Kark, Jeremy, 122
"Keep it up!," 208–10, 225
Keillor, Garrison, 151
Kennedy, John, Catholicism of, in
    campaign, 68
Khrushchev, Nikita, 29
King, Dana, 235–36
Koenig, Dr. Harold, 6, 60, 61, 63,
    73–74, 99–100, 104–5, 124, 128,
    136, 190, 197, 208–10, 225, 232,
    257, 258
    and colleagues, *Handbook of Religion
        and Health*, 6, 62, 127, 130–37,
        220, 232
    *The Healing Power of Faith*, 196–97
Korean War, 29
Kornhaber, Arthur, 124
Krucoff, Dr. Mitchell, 110–16, 165–68,
    172

laetrile, 188
*Lancet*, 117, 118, 166, 168, 257
Larimore, Dr. Walter, 4, 7, 63, 73, 124,
    198–201, 212–13

medicine (*continued*)
  journals of. *See* journals, medical
  popular vs. scientific, 19, 20
  rational, rise of, 22–26
  reporting on discoveries in, 65
  wrong beliefs held by, historically,
    74–75
medicines (drugs), testing efficacy of,
    41–42
meditation
  and blood pressure, 132
  neuroimaging of, 5
Medline, 78–80
meetings, professional, scientific
    findings announced at, 108
Mencken, H. L., 59, 214
mesothelioma, 88
metanarratives, 66
Miller, R. N., 133–34
miraculous healing, 21
monasteries, hospitals established by, 21
monastic life, and blood pressure, 132
Monitoring and Actualization of Noetic
    Trainings (MANTRA). *See*
    MANTRA studies
monotheism, 17
Mormons, health studies of, 76
mortality (or survival)
  attendance at church and, 82–83, 93,
    95, 140, 141–55
  as outcome, 165, 172
  religious involvement and, 151
Mueller, Dr. Paul, 74, 120–21, 138
multiple comparisons, 101–5
Muslims
  American, 226
  health studies of, 76
myocardial ischemia, 165
mystical experiences
  neurological basis of, 247–50
  reality of, claim, 249–50

National Aeronautics and Space
    Administration (NASA), 33
National Cancer Institute, 82
National Defense Education Act
    (NDEA), 32
National Institute for Healthcare
    Research (NIHR), 61–62

National Institutes of Health (NIH), 4,
    60, 61–62, 81
National Library of Medicine (NLM),
    78
National Science Foundation (NSF), 32,
    47
Nazi medical experiments, 201
Nease, Donald, 235
neurochemistry, religion as product of,
    243–45
neuroimaging, of meditation and prayer,
    5
neurotheology, 252
  new field of, 5, 246
neurotransmitters, 243–45
New Age movement, 11, 47, 51
Newberg, Dr. Andrew, 246–52
  and d'Aquili, "Why God Won't Go
    Away," 247
newborns, sleeping position of, 74–75
*New England Journal of Medicine,* 75,
    117, 118, 119
*Newsweek* magazine
  cover stories on religion and health,
    4, 7, 64–65, 246, 248
  Education Program Web site, 64
Newton, Isaac
  apple anecdote, 89
  *Principia,* 25–26
  revolutionary discoveries of, 174
New York Academy of Sciences, 8
*New Yorker* subscription, and Tay-Sachs
    disease, 96
*The New York Times,* 109
Nobel Prizes, American winners of, 33,
    125
noetic therapy, health outcomes of, 110,
    112–16
nonjudgmentalism, 48
nonlocal effects, 173–74
nonmaleficence ("do no harm"), 183

observation
  vs. authority, in discovering scientific
    truth, 23–26, 83
  systematic, in scientific research, 36,
    84–85, 89–88
observational studies, 43–45
  vs. clinical trials, 94–95

need for, 143–44
problems with, 45, 89–105, 144–47
O'Connor, Thomas, 10, 227
organ donation, religion and, 77
other factors than the key variable, effect
   on observational studies, 44
outcome variables, choice of, by
   experimenter (sharpshooter's
   fallacy), 172–73
Oxford University Press, 130

Pagán, José, 58
paperwork, in medical care, 57
*Parade* magazine, 7
paranormal phenomena, 49
   belief in, 49
Park, Robert, 97, 109, 176
Parliament of the World's Religions,
   114–15
patients
   autonomy of, as value, 195–96
   insensitive treatment of, 55–58
   powerlessness of, vis-a-vis doctors,
     13, 195
   questioning them about their faith, 4
   resistance to doctor's suggestions,
     203
   surveys of, as to religion-in-medicine,
     235–39
   treating them as whole people, 59
   unrealistic or unhealthy demands
     made by, 239
Pauly, Mark, 58
Peel, William, 198–201
peer-reviewed journals, 108
peptic ulcers, cause of, 74
physician-patient relationship, 13, 59,
   193–96
   asymmetry of, 194–95, 203
   goals of patient vs. those of doctor,
     202–3
physicians
   in ancient world, viewed as a calling,
     18, 21
   Christian, self-identified, 201–2
   disagreeing with, 204
   ethical abuses of, potentially, 13
   expertise of, confined to medicine,
     196, 211, 212

potential for manipulation and
   coercion by, 193–203
proselytizing by, 196–203
recommendations made to patients,
   153–54, 189–92
referral of spiritual matters to clergy,
   recommended, 266
as spiritual guides, patients' wishes as
   to, 235–39
as spiritual guides, suggested role,
   213–16, 226–28
time allocation of, and time spent
   with patients, 13, 216–20
training of, 220–23, 226, 228
pilot studies, 112
Pion, Georgine, 46
placebo, 37
Plante, Thomas, 6
Poles, 90
polio vaccine, 46
polytheism, 17
positron-emission tomography (PET),
   246
Posner, Dr. Gary, 66
possession by gods or spirits, 18
Powell, Dr. Lynda, 117–18, 120, 138,
   141–42, 147, 155
prayer
   as adjunct to standard medical care,
     172
   coerced by doctor, 203–4
   efficacy of, denominational
     differences in, proposed study of,
     168
   instead of medical care, 189
   intercessory. *See* intercessory prayer
   neuroimaging of, 5
   outside sources of ("noise"), 169–70
   power of, and kidnap case, 85–86
   of praise, vs. of petition, 204
   private, and health, 100
   quantification and specification of,
     170, 256–57
prediction, theory and, 175–76
preliterate societies, religion-medicine
   in, 16
press conferences, scientific findings
   announced at, 108–9
Presser, Stanley, 149, 234

some only remotely about religion, 78–80
religion-in-medicine
    brave new world of, and threats to scientific medicine, 4
    in Christian era, 21–22
    current status of, 65, 263–67
    demand for, question as to, 231–39
    ethical problems in, 9, 10, 181–206
    harm to religion from, 241–60
    history of, 11, 16–18
    impracticality of, 207–29
    patient demand for, questionable, 13–14
    popularity of, 8–10
    as satisfying form of human contact, 58–59
religiosity, quantification of, 253
religious conversion, recommended for health benefit, suggested, 182
religious density, 146–47
religious determinism (God's will), 188
religious freedom, 154, 195, 205
religious involvement
    and blood pressure, 104–5, 121–23, 127
    and cardiovascular disease, 127, 130–37
    and cardiovascular health, 133
    and health, 77, 100, 127–40, 189
    and heart transplants, 129
    measurement of, 242–43, 255
    and mortality, 151
    poll of, 6–7
    and weight control, 135–36
Renaissance, medicine in, 22–26
reports. See religion-and-health studies
research and development, federal funding of, 33
researchers, exaggerated claims of, as warning sign, 123–25
research proposals, 60–61
review papers, problems with, 120–21
risk ratio, 82
risky behavior, virginity pledges and, 109
rituals
    to cure illness, in preliterate societies, 16
    social acceptability of, 209–10

Rockville, Md., 61–62
Rodegast, Pat, 50
Romans, ancient, 11, 20
Rosenblum, Nancy, 209
Rosenthal, Robert, 39
Rosenthal effect, 39–41

The Saline Solution, 197–202
sample size, 38–39
satellites, Cold War competition of, 29–31
Scandinavians, 90
Scheurich, Dr. Neil, 9, 191
schoolchildren, intelligence testing of, and "blooming," 40–41
science
    advance of, in recent era, 27–28, 53
    called "linear" and "reductionist," 49
    differences from religion, 253–54, 264–65
    junk, voodoo, 97
    negative attitudes toward, in U.S., recently, 46, 49
    poor understanding of, by Americans, 47
    postmodernist critique of, 250–51
    revolutions in, 174–76
    support for, in Cold War, 31–33, 46–47
Science and Theology News, 61, 62–64
Science Citation Index, 117
science classes, evolutionary theory taught in, 36
scientific method, 12–13, 34–45, 242–43
    dissemination of results, 107–25
scientific truth, 252, 254
Scotch, Norman, 121–22
Scottish, 90
scurvy, vitamin C and, 171–72
secondary sources, 119
    problems with, 119–23
second opinion, 204
selective serotonin reuptake inhibitors (SSRIs), 245
self-fulfilling prophecy, 39
self-help movement, 47
self-presentation bias, 147–50, 233
self-selection, 45, 93–95, 144–47

serotonin
    and depression, 244–45
    and spiritual and religious
        inclinations, 243–45
Seventh-Day Adventists, health studies
    of, 76
sexuality, discussions of, with patients,
    192–93
sexually transmitted diseases (STDs), 192
    virginity pledges and, 109
shamans, 16
sharpshooter's fallacy, 97–104, 115, 131,
    172–73
Sherman, Allen, 6
skepticism, and scientific research, 48
Skrabanek, Petr, 214
Sloan, Richard (the author), 78, 130,
    162
Smart, Elizabeth, kidnap case, and
    prayer, 85–86
smoking
    health risks of, 82, 143–44, 153
    and longevity, 36
socioeconomic status, and health, 192
Sontag, Susan, "Illness as Metaphor,"
    184, 215
soul, fate of the, 21
sources, primary and secondary,
    119–23
*Southern Medical Journal,* 159
Soviet Union, in Cold War, 28–33
space program, 46
Spanish, 90
specialists, 57
SPECT technology, 246
spiritual history
    hypothetical counterexamples,
        209–12, 225
    impracticality of taking, 207–13,
        219–20
    ordinary history-taking as alternative
        to, 193
    questions suggested for, 190–91
    taking of, recommended to
        physicians, 4, 190, 197
    taking of, supportive and
        nonjudgmental manner of, 208–12
spirituality, "pop," 48

spontaneous remission, 37
sports
    and health, 191
    importance to some people,
        compared to religion, 191
*Sputnik,* effect on American psyche,
    29–31
standard medical care
    and cardiac treatment, 111
    prayer as adjunct to, 172
statistics, 38–39, 82, 92–105, 145
Stinson, Linda, 149, 234
stress-relaxation sessions, and cardiac
    treatment, 111
Study of the Therapeutic Effects of
    Intercessory Prayer (STEP), 61,
    168–69, 172
subjectivity, and irrationalism, 47–52
Sudden Infant Death Syndrome (SIDS),
    75
Sudsaung, Ratree, 131–32
Sulmasy, Dr. Daniel, 8
supernaturalism, 19
    recent increase in, 28, 48
surgery
    history of, 20, 23
    successes of, 54–55
Swyers, James, 62

Targ, Elisabeth, 98–99
Tay-Sachs disease, 96
Teller, Edward, 32
Templeton, Sir John, 60
terminal patients
    care of, 183
    religion and, 77
testing of hypotheses, 35
theory, and prediction, 175–76
therapeutics, beginning of, 23
Third International Mathematics and
    Science Study, 47
time use estimation, 149, 234
Titchener, Edward Bradford, 137
touch-therapy sessions, and cardiac
    treatment, 111
transcendental meditation (TM)
    and blood lipids, 132–33
    and reactivity, 133

treatment group, 143
treatment variables, 143, 144–45
Truman, Dr. John, 188
truth
    relativity of, 251
    religious, 251–52, 253–54
    scientific, 252, 254
Tyson, Neil deGrasse, 264

Union Theological Seminary, 226–27
United States
    in Cold War, 28–33
    ideal of freedom of, 205
    immigration policy, 90–92
    religious beliefs and practices, 6–7,
        231–34
    religious diversity in, 226, 254–55
    student performance, compared to
        other countries', 47
Unity School of Christianity, 111
University of Minnesota, Center for
    Spirituality & Healing, 5
University of North Dakota, School of
    Medicine and Health Sciences, 5
U.S. Army, intelligence testing by, 90
USA Today, 7, 66
U.S. News & World Report, 7, 67
U.S. Preventive Services Task Force
    (USPSTF), 216–18

Vanderpool, Dr. Harold, 121–23
variables
    primary vs. confounding, 144–47

treatment (causal, primary, key) and
    outcome, 143, 144–45
Vesalius, 23
    De Humani Corporis Fabrica, 23
victim, blaming the, 184–87
virginity pledges, and STDs and lower
    risky behavior, 109
Virtue, Doreen, 6, 248
    Angel Medicine, 49–50
visions, seeing, and hearing voices, 248
vitalism, 27–28
vitamin C, and scurvy, 171–72
vitamins, health claims for, 84
voodoo science, 97

Wadland, Dr. William, 235
Wall Street Journal, 67
Washington County, Maryland, 82
The Washington Post, 7, 113–15
weight control, religious involvement
    and, 135–36
weighting, 162–64
Weinberg, Steven, 8
Wenneberg, Stig, 133
Western Europe, religion in, 232–33
Western Journal of Medicine, 98–99
Wills, Gary, 205
Wilson, Dr. William, 63
workshops, on enlightenment, 50–51
World Values Survey, 232

yeshiva education, and blood pressure,
    122–23